Critical Care

14: Updates in Outreach, Cardiology, Neuroscience and Trauma

Edited by
DR SAXON RIDLEY
Consultant in Anaesthesia and Intensive Care
Glan Clwyd Hospital
Sarn Lane, Rhyl
Denbighshire, LL18 5UJ

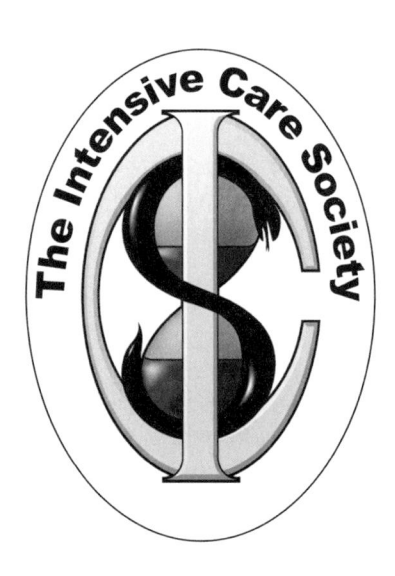

Published by
The Intensive Care Society
Churchill House
35 Red Lion Square
London WC1R 4SG

Copyright @ The Intensive Care Society

Printed by
Latimer Trend & Company Ltd
Estover Road
Plymouth PL6 7PY

First Published 2008

ISBN 978-0-9555897-1-3

Available from the Intensive Care Society
Tel +44 (0)20 7280 4350
Fax +44(0)20 7280 4369
Email: pauline@ics.ac.uk
Web: http://www.ics.ac.uk

Price: £14.99

Contents

Contributors   4
Introduction   6

1. Outreach – Does it help?   10
   DR PAUL HOLDER and DR BRIAN CUTHBERTSON
2. Validating Track and Trigger Scores   19
   DR DAVID GOLDHILL
3. Myocardial ischaemia; when to intervene   28
   DR ROBERT SAPSFORD
4. Echocardiography in the Intensive Care Unit   45
   DR SEAN BENNETT
5. Biomarkers in Acute Coronary Syndrome –   58
   Introducing Heart-Fatty Acid-Binding Protein (H-FABP)
   DR NIAMH KILCULLEN and PROF ALISTAIR HALL
6. Evidence based review in Neurosciences: Management of Head Injury   75
   DR STEPHEN WILSON, DR PAUL MURPHY and PROF MARK BELLAMY
7. Head injury: The Lund Approach   94
   PROF CARL-HENRIK NORDSTRÖM
8. Temperature Reduction after Acute Brain injury   109
   DR MANOJ SAXENA, PROF PETER ANDREWS, MS BRIDGET HARRIS and DR OLAV THULESIUS
9. Musculoskeletal disorders in ICU   118
   DR JOHN MOORE and DANIEL CONWAY
10. The London Bombings, July 7th 2005   130
    DR HUGH MONTGOMERY
11. Trauma outcome: Is it all in the genes?   137
    PROF PETER GIANNOUDIS and DR STATHIS KATSOULIS
12. Low Volume versus High Volume Resuscitation in Trauma   181
    PROF MONTY MYTHEN

Contributors

Prof Peter JD Andrews, MD, MB ChB, FRCA
Intensive Care Unit, Western General Hospital, Crewe Road South, Edinburgh, EH4 2XU, UK

Prof Mark C Bellamy, MA, FRCA
Intensive Care Unit, St James's University Hospital, Leeds, LS9 7TF, UK

Dr Sean Bennett, FRCA
Intensive Carte Unit, Castle Hill Hospital, Castle Road, Hull, HU16 5JQ, UK

Dr Daniel Conway, FRCA
Critical Care Unit, Manchester Royal Infirmary, Oxford Road, Manchester, M13 9WL, UK

Brian H Cuthbertson, MB ChB, FRCA, MD
Health Services Research Unit, Polwarth Building, University of Aberdeen, Foresterhill, Aberdeen, Scotland, AB25 2ZD, UK

Prof Peter V Giannoudis, BSC, MB, MD, EEC (Ortho)
Department of Trauma & Orthopaedics, St James' University Hospital, Beckett Street, Leeds, LS9 7TF, UK

Dr David Goldhill, MA, MBBS, FRCA, MD, EDIC
Royal Orthopaedic Hospital, Stanmore, Middlesex, HA7 4LP, UK

Professor Alistair Hall, PhD, FRCP
Department of Cardiology, Leeds General Infirmary, Leeds, LS1 3EX, UK

Ms Bridget Harris, RGN, DipN, Msc
University of Edinburgh & Western General Hospital, Crewe Road South, Edinburgh, EH4 2XU, UK

Paul Holder, MB ChB, FRCA
Intensive Care Unit, Aberdeen Royal Infirmary, Westburn Road, Aberdeen, Scotland, AB25 2ZN, UK

Dr Stathis Katsoulis, MRCS
Department of Trauma & Orthopaedics, St James' University Hospital, Beckett Street, Leeds, LS9 7TF, UK

Dr Niamh Kilcullen, MRCP
Department of Cardiology, Leeds General Infirmary, Leeds, LS1 3EX, UK

Dr Hugh Montgomery, MB BS, BSc, MD, MRCP
University College London Hospitals, Middlesex Hospital, Mortimer Street, London, WC1E 6JJ, UK

Dr John Moore, FRCA, MRCP
Critical Care Unit, Manchester Royal Infirmary, Oxford Road, Manchester, M13 9WL, UK

Dr Paul Murphy, FRCA
Neuro Intensive Care Unit, Leeds General Infirmary, Leeds, LS1 3EX, UK

Prof Michael (Monty) Mythen, MD, MRCP, FRCA
University College London, Head of The Portex Anaesthesia, Intensive Care and Respiratory Unit, Institute of Child Health, London WC1N 1EH, UK

Prof Carl-Henrik Nordström, MD, PhD
Department of Neurosurgery, Lund University Hospital, SE-221 85, Lund, Sweden

Dr Robert Sapsford, BSc, MD, FRCP
Department of Cardiology, Level 4 Gledhow Wing, St James's University Hospital, Beckett Street, Leeds, LS9 7TF, UK

Dr Manoj Saxena, MBBS, MRCP, FJFICM
Intensive Care Unit, Western General Hospital, Crewe Road South, Edinburgh, EH4 2XU, UK

Prof Olav Thulesius, MD, PhD
Department of Clinical Physiology, Faculty of Medicine, University Hospital Linkoping, Sweden

Dr Stephen J Wilson, MRCP, FRCA
Academic Unit of Anaesthesia, James's University Hospital, Leeds, LS9 7TF, UK

Introduction

Updates in Outreach, Cardiology, Neuroscience and Trauma
This, the fourteenth volume in the Critical Care Focus series, offers updates in four topical areas of critical care. The chapters are based upon the lectures delivered by the authors at The Intensive Care Society's Spring Meeting held in May 2006. The lectures were delivered by internationally renowned experts. Their clear description of important current issues will enable critical care practitioners to offer appropriate options to the patients and their relatives.

Outreach – Does it help?
Doctors Holder and Cuthbertson present the case of need for outreach teams and review the evidence for their beneficial effects. Although the outreach concept seems intuitively sensible, the reviewed studies fail to demonstrate a consistent effect in terms of reduced rates of cardiac arrest or mortality. The authors make the point that the positive effect of education on the recognition and prompt management of unstable patients may have been overlooked in these studies and that track and trigger scoring systems are a key component of such education.

Validating Track and Trigger Scores
Abnormal physiological values are associated with adverse outcome and there is much sense, as well as precedent, in basing track and trigger systems on these measurements. Dr Goldhill points out that improving outcome requires the physiological data to be collected accurately and with sufficient frequency. The basis for the track and trigger systems used in UK hospitals is reviewed. However if a response is triggered, it must be capable of altering outcome delivering staff with skills, training and experience with the essential equipment, resources and support to the deteriorating patient.

Myocardial ischaemia; when to intervene
Dr Sapsford reviews the interpretation of cardiac biomarkers (troponins) and other recent developments in the management of acute coronary syndrome in the critically ill. Peri-operative ischaemia is frequently the trigger for organ dysfunction requiring intensive care support. Dr Sapsford discusses how best to interpret troponin levels before describing the pathophysiology of plaque rupture and the critical care management of acute coronary syndrome.

Echocardiography in the Intensive Care Unit
Dr Bennett compares transthoracic and transoesophageal echocardiography. Although transthoracic echocardiography is dependent upon the quality of the acoustic window, it is probably the most useful type. However, there are certain circumstances (usually structural abnormalities of the heart and aorta) where transoesophageal echocardiography is needed. Despite the limited number of class 1 indications, echocardiography on the ICU is useful for assessment and optimisation of cardiac function (including deriving functional measures), chest trauma, systemic embolism, aortic dissection and other structural pathologies. Dr Bennett illustrated most of these with colour images.

Biomarkers in Acute Coronary Syndrome –Introducing Heart-Fatty Acid-Binding Protein (H-FABP)
Dr Kilcullen and Prof Hall review the history and efficacy of biomarkers for detecting cardiac ischaemia. Heart-fatty acid-binding protein is one of a group of low molecular weight proteins involved in lipid homeostasis; it is released from the cytosol following myocardial ischaemia. Therefore heart-fatty acid-binding protein might be a useful biomarker especially as it peaks quickly at 6 to 8 hours and returns to normal levels by 24 hours. The authors review studies demonstrating the potential value of this new marker of myocardial ischaemia.

Evidence based review in Neurosciences: Management of Head Injury
The authors make the point that despite the large number of clinical trials in neurosurgical critical care, there are remarkably few guidelines that can be supported by high quality scientific research. Therefore the aim of their review is to summarise and condense the relevant issues from the European Brain Injury Consortium and Brain Trauma Foundation guidelines, the Cochrane Collaboration reports and the other independent reviewers. Using these sources the authors provide some simple answers to clinical questions about treating the severely brain injured patient. These answers will be useful for those clinicians treating brain injured patients outside the neurosurgical unit.

Head injury: the Lund approach
Prof Nordström outlines the two apparently incompatible principles for reducing increased intracranial pressure in severe head injury. According to US guidelines reducing dangerous increases in ICP can be achieved by increasing mean arterial blood pressure and cerebral perfusion pressure. A contradictory view was presented from Lund suggesting that reducing ICP can be achieved by a pharmacologically

induced decrease in mean arterial blood pressure and cerebral perfusion pressure. It seems highly unlikely both of these hypotheses are true. Prof Nordstrom examines the physiological and biochemical foundations of the two conflicting principles.

Temperature Reduction after Acute Brain injury
The authors review the current evidence for temperature reduction after neuronal injury. They attempt to answer two important questions. First, can mild systemic hypothermia improve clinical outcomes if applied within the first few minutes after injury and second does avoiding pyrexia in the days after injury reduce disability? Unfortunately there appears to be no clinical data from randomised trials to support the mild hypothermia in the conditions most commonly seen in adult critical care but physical cooling techniques and drug therapy reversing pyrexia may be beneficial. Most importantly the authors confirm that further evaluation is required.

Musculoskeletal disorders in ICU
Musculoskeletal disorders are frequently associated with critical illness. Drs Moore and Conway describe the pathophysiology of critical illness polyneuropathy and myopathy as well as outlining how to differentiate between the two conditions. The authors emphasise the importance of prevention (avoiding risk factors) and aiding recovery through a structured rehabilitation programme.

The London Bombings, July 7th 2005
Dr Montgomery outlines the classification of injuries sustained after explosions and summarizes the history of previous terrorist attacks on London. Details of the attacks on the 7th July are discussed as well as how and where the casualties were treated. The mortality rate is compared to other recent attacks. The specific problems faced by hospitals and intensive care units in particular are reviewed.

Trauma outcome: Is it all in the genes?
Professor Giannoudis and Dr Katsoulis describe the relationship between genetic configuration and disease; they focus particularly on trauma and surgery. The authors describe how changes in genetic material may affect the immune response and hence our predisposition to disease processes and complications. They concentrate on how genetic polymorphisms produce their effects in sepsis by altering cytokines, receptors, binding proteins and other inflammation - related proteins. Although quite technical, the chapter introduces simple genetic terms and usefully describes these in a glossary at the end of the chapter.

Low Volume versus High Volume Resuscitation in Trauma:
Prof Mythen describes the limited evidence supporting the use of isotonic crystalloids in early resuscitation before going on to discuss the advantages and disadvantages of the different fluids that could be used in the hospital setting. Prof Mythen emphasises the importance of surgical control of haemorrhage and the difference in strategies required if the injuries include a head injury.

1: Outreach – Does it help?

DRS PAUL HOLDER and BRIAN CUTHBERTSON

Introduction
As in all other specialities, critical care is searching for ways to improve patient outcomes whilst more effectively utilising resources. The organisation of critical care units has previously centralised patients with the greatest need and then devoted significant resources to that area. A new approach to care of the critically ill has been suggested; this involves the transit of skills and knowledge out to the general ward environment in an attempt to prevent patients deteriorating. If intensive care unit (ICU) admission is required then it should be expedited to ensure that the patient is exposed to the minimum risk and the best possible outcome achieved. Such an approach would also provide an increased level of care on the general ward to where critical care patients could be discharged safely. This concept is referred to as outreach.

The idea of critical care outreach has been widely promoted. The original Medical Emergency Team (MET) concept was developed in Liverpool, New South Wales, in 1989 and has been widely introduced in Australian hospitals since the 1990s. The MET concept involves senior medical and nursing critical care staff being called by any member of the hospital staff when a certain set of physiological parameters are breached or when there is concern for a deteriorating patient [1] (Table 1).

More recently political and clinical enthusiasm for outreach has led to widespread introduction of outreach teams in the NHS in England, though notably not in other parts of the UK. In 1999 the Audit commission report entitled 'Critical to success' recommended as a high priority that acute hospitals should develop an outreach service to support ward staff in managing patients at risk [2]. The Department of Health further supported this with the publication of 'Comprehensive Critical Care' which recommended that outreach become an integral part of each trust's critical care services [3]. The report stated that outreach has three key aims:
  1) to avert ICU admissions (or assure that ICU admission is timely by identifying deteriorating patients)
  2) to enable ICU discharges
  3) to share critical care skills.

The composition of the outreach team should be multi-disciplinary and led by a qualified critical care clinician, though the report does not

Table 1. Medical emergency team calling criteria [13].

Airway
    If threatened
Breathing
    All respiratory arrests
    Respiratory rate <5 breaths per minute
    Respiratory rate >36 breaths per minute
Circulation
    All cardiac arrests
    Pulse rate <40 beats per minute
    Pulse rate >140 beats per minute
    Systolic blood pressure <90 mmHg
Neurology
    Sudden fall in level of consciousness (fall in GCS of >2 points)
    Repeated or extended seizures
Other
    Any patient you are worried about that does not fit the above criteria

state that this clinician should be a doctor, which is in contrast to the MET approach. These recommendations were funded centrally to facilitate such service developments.

'Critical Care Outreach 2003: Progress in developing services' highlighted outreach's key principles, yet noted that outreach delivery was variable across the country. The report highlighted some of the major problems of outreach as implemented in the UK. The authors noted the significant variability in delivery and organisation of outreach and that dedicated funding is required for implementation. The report stated that further research and evaluation are required to identify the most effective configurations for outreach teams and advocated track and trigger systems as a core component. Unfortunately, there is no clear evidence to support the use of any individual track and trigger system and so the use of individualised systems in different hospitals causes confusion [4].

In 2005, the National Confidential Enquiry into Patient Outcome and Death (NCEPOD) published the report called 'An acute problem?' examining the care of acute medical ICU admissions [5]. Surprisingly given the national move towards outreach, the report stated that 27% of hospitals did not use an early warning system, and that 44% of hospitals did not provide an outreach service; where outreach was developed, the times of availability were not stated. The report recommended that each hospital should use a track and trigger system. Furthermore although this recommendation was not based on any findings within the report, NCEPOD echoed other bodies in encouraging hospitals to provide formal outreach services available 24 hours per day seven days per week. However despite the use of early warning scoring systems and outreach teams in the majority of audited hospitals, the hospitals in the report failed to show any improvements in early recognition and intervention in acutely unwell patients. There was no difference between those hospitals with and without outreach in the appropriateness or timeliness of admission to ICU, nor indeed in mortality.

The fact that so many hospitals do not have outreach seems surprising given that it is seen as a clinically intuitive concept and the well established need for improvement. Also the large numbers of national bodies that have supported the principles of outreach must further add to the pressure to adopt the system. Interestingly, the Scottish and Welsh health departments did not endorse outreach and thus there is neither the same pressure nor incentive to change in these countries. One possible reason for this apparent inertia may be the lack of evidence demonstrating clear benefit or a lack of funding.

The evidence
Buist *et al.* reported a non-randomised, population based study of before and after the introduction of a MET into a teaching hospital [6]. They demonstrated a significant decrease in the incidence of and mortality from unexpected cardiac arrests, odds ratio 0.5 (95% Confidence Interval (CI): 0.35 - 0.73). This seemed to be largely due to the fact that they expected more cardiac arrests and placed more appropriate do-not-resuscitate orders. The study also showed an increase in unplanned admissions to ICU after the introduction of the MET (although the statistical significance of this result is not stated). One problem raised by the authors was that the control and study periods were separated by three years.

Ball *et al.* published the results of a non-randomised population based study, in which they compared historical controls with patients cared for by a nurse only outreach team, which was available for 12 hours each day [7]. The operational policy of this team appeared to be limited to those patients who had been discharged from ICU rather than including other acutely ill patients. After the introduction of the outreach team, there was a significant increase in survival to hospital discharge (risk ratio 1.08 (95% CI: 1.00 - 1.18)) and a significant decrease in ICU re-admission rate (risk ratio 0.48 (95% CI: 0.26 -

0.87)); however this decrease in re-admission rate only returned the unit to the national average. Garcea *et al.* published a retrospective observational study, comparing before and after introduction of outreach to surgical wards [8]. The team comprised two senior nurses and a nurse consultant; the service had an ICU consultant as the lead clinician whose level of involvement was not defined. The team's original remit involved the follow up of critical care discharges and education concentrating on recognition of the sick patient; however this was later expanded to include the direct referral of patients highlighted by an early warning scoring system. They tentatively concluded that outreach teams may have a favourable impact on mortality rate amongst re-admissions to critical care. Critical care mortality before outreach was 14.3% and fell to 9.8% afterwards while in-hospital mortality fell 9.3% to 4.8%.

Bellomo *et al.* performed a prospective, controlled before and after trial to examine introducing an ICU based MET in a large teaching hospital [9]. The team evaluated and treated any patient who was deemed to be at risk of developing an adverse outcome by nursing, paramedical or medical staff. The authors concluded that the introduction of the MET was associated with a significant reduction in the number of adverse events (relative risk reduction 57.8%, $p<0.001$), post-operative mortality (relative risk reduction 36.6%, p= 0.018) and mean duration of hospital stay (from 23.8 to 18.9 days, p= 0.009). Thus they suggested that the MET was associated with major cost savings and increased efficiency of hospital care, with an estimated decrease in hospital stay of nearly 12000 bed days per year. The authors noted that the decrease in adverse events was only partly accounted for by the interventions of the MET and that the increased awareness of the significance and consequences of physiological instability brought about by the MET improved care. The implication that education was an important factor seems to have been somewhat overlooked.

Leary and Ridley examined the effects of an outreach service on ICU re-admissions to ICU by comparing the numbers and reasons for re-admission before and after the introduction of outreach in their hospital [10]. Their study could not detect changes in numbers or reasons for re-admissions; the authors stated that other parameters should be used to examine the effectiveness of the outreach service, despite reducing the re-admission rate being one of the highlighted aims of outreach. Bristow *et al.* published a prospective cohort comparison of three similarly sized public hospitals [11]. At Hospital 1, the cardiac arrest team was replaced by a MET while at Hospitals 2 and 3, the arrest team operated as previously. Adjustment was made for case-mix between hospitals. The results showed that the MET hospital had fewer unanticipated critical care admissions after adjustment, mainly due to the fact that they anticipated more admissions. Hospital 2 had 49 (95% CI: 20 - 87) more unanticipated critical care admissions over a six-month period, and Hospital 3 had 92 (95% CI: 47 - 146) more, compared with Hospital 1. However, there was no difference in either the in-hospital cardiac arrest rate or total death rate.

Preistley *et al.* performed a ward cluster randomised trial of the phased introduction of critical care outreach to a general hospital [12]. A nurse consultant led their team supported by experienced nurses providing 24-hour cover. Ward staff used a locally devised patient at risk scoring system to trigger referral. This study found a significant reduction in hospital mortality in wards where the service operated compared to those where it did not (odds ratio 0.52 (95% CI: 0.32 – 0.85)). Analysis of whether outreach increased the length of hospital stay was equivocal, and data on cardiac arrest rate, overall hospital mortality, do not resuscitate orders and ICU admissions were not included. Importantly they also appear to demonstrate improved outcome related to the pre-intervention educational programme.

The MERIT study represents the best available evidence of the effect of outreach and recruited more patients than all other studies combined into a randomised trial [13]. In this study, large Australian hospitals with an ICU and emergency department that did not use the MET system were identified and offered the opportunity to participate in the study. The 23 hospitals that agreed to participate were randomised to receive standardised MET implementation (n = 12) or to be controls (n = 11) and thus operate entirely as previously with no indication that a study was being undertaken. Over a period of four months, an educational strategy was undertaken to prepare the study hospitals for the introduction of the MET. This included educating staff about calling criteria, identifying the patient at risk and the importance of rapidly calling the MET should any of the calling criteria be fulfilled. After MET implementation was complete, an impressive system of reminders was issued to ensure that calling criteria were not forgotten or overlooked. The study protocol required that the MET should be at least the equivalent of the pre-existing cardiac arrest team with at least one doctor and a nurse from the emergency department or ICU. The study showed that the MET system did not significantly reduce any of the study outcomes: cardiac arrest (odds ratio 0.94 (95% CI: 0.79 – 1.13)); unexpected death (odds ratio 1.03 (95% CI: 0.84 – 1.28)) or unplanned ICU admission (odds ratio 1.04 (95% CI: 0.89 – 1.21)). However, the authors point out three main flaws in their study's ability to disprove the null hypothesis. Firstly, they suggest that the six-month study period was inadequate as the study was underpowered. However, the very small difference in the incidence of the primary outcome measure between groups suggests that even if they did continue, the number needed to treat to prevent one combined outcome would be approximately 2000. Secondly, in the control hospitals the cardiac arrest teams are often called to critically ill patients who have not yet suffered a cardiac arrest and thus are acting as informal METs. This is countered by the fact that far more MET calls were made in the intervention hospitals compared to controls although many calls were inappropriate. Finally, the study demonstrated that even in MET hospitals documentation and responses to changes in vital signs were not adequate despite an educational programme. The authors did not comment that the trial demonstrated that the MET calling system failed to allow early recognition and intervention in their patients as they failed to see half of the appropriate ICU referrals before their admission and failed to identify the majority of patients more than 15 minutes before a cardiac arrest. They also did not highlight the fact that the only significant improvement in trial outcomes was related to the pre-intervention educational programme. The finding that education could improve outcome from critical illness is indeed a major finding and should be given great emphasis. It would be far more cost-effective to educate staff than to provide 24-hour outreach cover.

Summary of evidence
The nature of outreach makes studies evaluating its effectiveness difficult and expensive. As a result most of the available evidence is methodologically flawed and represents at best level 2 evidence [14]. The obvious exception is the MERIT study, which failed to demonstrate an improved outcome. A further problem with the evidence base is the heterogeneity of studied interventions. Whilst a significant difference with one type of service can be demonstrated, it is not known how transferable the results might be in different clinical circumstances. The current evidence does show a balance between supporting some aspects of outreach and showing no benefit in others. On this basis the full implementation of outreach in its current form probably cannot be promoted as evidence based.

The way forward
Whilst the beneficial effects of outreach have not been clearly proven, the previous system of patient care was failing some acutely unwell patients. There is no doubt that a large number of preventable adverse events are preceded by a detectable period of physiological instability [15]. The recognition and documentation of warning signs and events

is inadequate [16,17] and as demand for healthcare increases, this situation may worsen. The traditional response to an emergency is frequently inadequate because of nursing staff who record continuing deterioration without directly intervening, junior medical staff who have little formal training in resuscitation of the critically ill and senior medical staff who do not have sufficient opportunity to maintain their knowledge and resuscitation skills. Unfortunately the current pattern of medical consultants working has also been shown to be failing patients, in that they are not always available to attend their sickest patients [5].

Part of the solution is ensuring that the deteriorating patient is recognised as early as possible. The current recommendations are that track and trigger systems should be used in all clinical areas to identify the failing patient. However there is no system that has been demonstrated to be universally appropriate and as a result different systems are used in different hospitals and they are poorly applied. If a system could reliably identify the deteriorating patient at an early stage, then this should become a national standard, and taught early on in all medical, nursing and paramedical curricula. This early introduction and re-iteration during both training and later career would highlight the importance of identifying quickly the patients in need. Furthermore if the system is standardised then a national audit could be undertaken to highlight areas of potential improvement.

The basic skills such as airway protection, appropriate use of oxygen therapy, fluid resuscitation and also recognising the need for higher levels of care must also be addressed. These skills are more commonly used in critical care so it would seem appropriate that critical care staff disperse these skills through the rest of the hospital by formal education and staff rotation. The application of outreach should be most appropriate when both medical and nursing staffing levels are at their lowest (i.e. outside of normal working hours). Therefore if outreach is to be most effective, it should probably be available at all times but the impact of such a change should be carefully studied. The composition of outreach teams should be examined in more detail. A truly multi-disciplinary approach may be beneficial, with senior physicians and nurses being included. Again the benefits of specific outreach team composition have not been studied but is important as including senior personnel would represent a major resource issue.

Previously, on-call commitment allowed junior doctors to gain experience in the identification, assessment and immediate management of the acutely unwell patient without the direct input of senior staff. These work practices clearly failed our sickest patients.

With the advent of the hospital-at-night team, learning experience will be further diluted. Therefore existing outreach teams should include junior staff from all specialities because education is the only intervention that has been shown to improve outcome [9, 13].

References
1. Lee A, Bishop G, Hillman K, Daffurn K. The medical emergency team. Anaesthesia and Intensive Care 1995; 23: 183-186.
2. Audit Commission. Critical to Success - The place of efficient and effective critical care services within the acute hospital. London: Audit Commission, 1999. http://www.audit-commission.gov.uk/Products/NATIONAL-REPORT/40B50F26-ED9F-4317-A056-042B31AEA454/CriticalToSuccess.pdf.
3. Comprehensive Critical care: a review of adult critical care services. London: Department of Health, 2000. http://www.dh.gov.uk/assetRoot/04/08/28/72/04082872.pdf.
4. The National Outreach Report 2003. Critical Care Outreach 2003: Progress in Developing Services. London: Department of Health and Modernisation Agency, 2003. http://www.modern.nhs.uk/criticalcare/5021/7117/78001-DoH-CareOutreach.pdf.
5. An acute problem? The National Confidential Enquiry into Patient Outcome and Death. London: NCEPOD, 2005. http://www.ncepod.org.uk/2005.htm.
6. Buist MD, Moore GE, Bernard SA, *et al.* Effects of a medical emergency team on reduction of incidence of and mortality from unexpected cardiac arrests in hospital: preliminary study. British Medical Journal 2002; 324: 387-390.
7. Ball C, Kirby K, Williams S. Effect of the critical care outreach team on patient survival to discharge from hospital and readmission to critical care: non-randomised population based study. British Medical Journal 2003; 327: 1014-1017.
8. Garcea G, Thomasset S, McClelland L, *et al.* Impact of a critical care outreach team on critical care readmissions and mortality. Acta Anaesthesiologica Scandanavica 2004; 48: 1096-1100.
9. Bellomo R, Goldsmith D, Uchino S, *et al.* Prospective controlled trial of medical emergency team on postoperative morbidity and mortality rates. Critical Care Medicine 2004; 32: 916-921.
10. Leary T, Ridley S. Impact of an outreach team on re-admissions to a critical care unit. Anaesthesia 2003; 58: 328-332.
11. Bristow PJ, Hilman KM, Chey T, *et al.* Rate of in-hospital arrest, deaths and intensive care admissions: the affect of a medical emergency team. Medical Journal of Australia 2000; 173: 236-240.

12. Preistly G, Watson W, Rashidian A, *et al.* Introducing critical care Outreach: a ward-randomised trial of phased introduction in a general hospital. Intensive Care Medicine 2004; 30: 1398-1404.
13. MERIT study investigators. Introduction of the medical emergency team (MET) system: a cluster randomised trial. Lancet 2005; 365: 2091-2097.
14. Harbour R, Miller J. A new system for grading recommendations in evidence based medicine. British Medical Journal 2001; 323: 334-336.
15. Schein R, Hazday N, Pena M, *et al.* Clinical antecedents to in-hospital cardiopulmonary arrest. Chest 1990; 98: 1388-1391.
16. Garrard C, Young D. Suboptimal care of patients before admission to intensive care. British Medical Journal 1998; 316: 1841-1842.
17. McGloin H, Adam S, Singer M. The quality of pre-ICU care influences outcome of patients admitted from the ward. Clinical Intensive Care 1997; 8: 104.

2: Validating Track and Trigger Scores

DR DAVID GOLDHILL

What are Track and Trigger Scores
Track and trigger is the term given to scoring systems designed to identify and monitor ward patients who are, or who may become, critically ill. All track and trigger systems are based around abnormal physiological values, although softer indications such as 'concern' or 'shortness of breath' may also initiate a response. Increasing scores or marked abnormality in any physiological parameter will identify patients at risk. Repeated measurement of the score provides a method of following improvement or deterioration in the patient's physiology. Inherent in these scoring systems is a trigger that initiates a response at a predefined score or other threshold. These systems will therefore track patients and trigger a response with the aim of improving outcome.

Physiological abnormality and outcome
Physiological abnormality is associated with adverse outcome. Abnormal physiology is the basis of all major intensive care outcome prediction models such as APACHE, SAPS and MPM for predicting mortality and morbidity [1-3]. The majority of patients who suffer a cardiorespiratory arrest in hospital have abnormal physiological values recorded in the hours before the arrest [4-6]. Similarly patients who die on hospital wards have documented abnormal physiology in the hours preceding death [7,8]. A high percentage of patients admitted from hospital wards to the intensive care unit (ICU) have abnormal physiology in the hours before admission [9,10]. The greater the number of physiological abnormalities recorded from patients on hospital wards the higher their mortality [11,12]. Furthermore, the longer patients are in hospital on a ward before admission to ICU the more deranged their physiological values and the more likely they are to die [13]. However, abnormal physiological values may not be the only, or even the best, way of identifying high risk patients. Patients may suffer an adverse event without premonitory physiological signs. However, patients admitted to a hospital ward are already selected because of illness, need for an operation or other procedure. It will be rare for them to die, require cardiopulmonary resuscitation or be admitted to ICU as an emergency without abnormal physiological values.

CRITICAL CARE FOCUS 14: UPDATES

Measuring physiological values

Routine physiological measurements undertaken on the ward typically consist of temperature, heart rate, blood pressure, respiratory rate, oxygen saturation and an assessment of level of consciousness. Some of these measurements are less intrusive and easier to take than others. Fluid balance may also be important although accurate urinary output is generally only possible in a catheterised patient. Perhaps surprisingly the respiratory rate is often the worst recorded [14]. This may be because there is no reliable monitor that will accurately measure it and in clinical practice it can be quite difficult and relatively time consuming to accurately record the number of breaths taken. By contrast measurement of oxygen saturation is simple and does not disturb the patient. It should be remembered that until fairly recently equipment routinely measuring this parameter was not available on the wards. Measures of arterial blood pressure may be intermittent and may disturb or wake the patient. Similarly assessment of level of consciousness disturbs the patient. It is possible that equipment development will allow better measurement of some of these parameters or that other measures may prove to be useful in the future. Possible candidates for this would include muscle oxygen tension, regional blood flow, circulating blood volume, lactate concentration and acid base status.

Table 1. The MET calling criteria described by Buist *et al.* [25]

Airway	Respiratory distress
	Threatened airway
Breathing	Respiratory rate < 6 or > 30 breaths per minute
Peripheral oxygen saturation	< 90% on O_2
	Difficulty speaking
Circulation	Systolic arterial pressure < 90 mmHg despite treatment
	Heart rate > 130 beats per minute
Neurology	Unexplained decreased in conscious level
	Agitation / delirium
	Repeated / prolonged seizures
Others	Concern about patient
	Uncontrolled pain
	Failure to respond to treatment
	Unable to obtain prompt help

Although there is an established link between abnormal physiology and adverse outcome, many studies have demonstrated that measurements are commonly not recorded in the hours before an adverse event [15,16]. The reasons for this may relate to lack of equipment and its inadequacies, or ward staff who do not make the decision to record values with the necessary frequency or accuracy, or who do not have the time and training to perform these tasks. Action to call medical emergency teams (MET) appears to be more likely around the time of shift handover or when physiological measurements are made [17]. Even when measurements are made and abnormal values recorded, the appropriate team may not be called [16].

Examples of track and trigger scores
METs were introduced in Liverpool, New South Wales in 1989 [18]. They were designed to respond to single measures of deranged physiology or concern by ward staff. Several examples of MET calling criteria have been published with a variety of different criteria for triggering a response (Table 1). Morgan in 1997 first described a physiologically-based early warning score (EWS) designed to identify critically ill ward patients [19]. This score incorporated heart rate, systolic blood pressure, respiratory rate, temperature and an assessment of level of consciousness (Table 2). Variations of the

Table 2. Early Warning Score (EWS) originally published by Morgan *et al* [19] A: alert, V: responds to voice, P: responds to pain, U: unresponsive.

Score	3	2	1	0	1	2	3
Heart rate; beats per minute		=40	41-50	51-100	101-110	111-130	=130
Systolic blood pressure; mmHg	≤70	71-80	81-100	101-199		=200	
Respiratory rate; breaths per minute		≤8		9-14	15-20	21-29	=30
Temperature; °C		=35	35.1-36.5	36.6-37.4	=37.5		
Central nervous system				A	V	P	U

EWS or the Modified Early Warning system (MEWS) are commonly used as scoring systems in the UK. In the original EWS, the subjectively defined 'normal' range was awarded zero points with up to three points given for increasingly abnormal physiology. The individual scores are summed to give a total score. In commonly used early warning scores, triggers are based on this score, a high score in a single parameter or some other combination.

Table 3. Classification of track and trigger warning systems. Definitions taken from *The National Outreach Report 2003*. Department of Health and National Health Service Modernisation Agency, 2003 [20].

Single parameter systems
Tracking: periodic observation of selected basic signs
Trigger: one or more extreme observational values

Multiple parameter systems
Tracking: periodic observation of selected basic vital signs
Trigger: two or more extreme observational values

Aggregate weighted scoring systems
Tracking: periodic observation of selected basic vital signs and the assignment of weighted scores to physiological values with calculation of a total score
Trigger: achieving a previously agreed trigger threshold with the total score

Combination systems
Elements of single or multiple parameter systems in combination with aggregate weighted scoring

Over the years many variations and developments of early warning scores have been described. They incorporate different combinations of physiological parameters and a wide range of scoring systems and trigger thresholds. They can be broadly summarised as single parameter or multiple parameter systems, aggregate weighted scoring systems or combinations [20] (Table 3). A recent review by the Intensive Care Audit and Research Centre (ICNARC) [21] found 35 papers describing a track and trigger tool. In total, 25 tools are described of which 13 are single parameter systems, one multiple parameter system and 11 aggregate scoring systems. These systems are known by an array of acronyms including MEWS, PAR, HOT, S.E.C.S., Condition C, PERT, DMEWS, MMEWS, PARS, EWSS and PAR-T.

A whole systems approach
If track and trigger systems are to alter outcome, several elements must work successfully together. Firstly physiological measurements must be made. They must be the correct parameters capable of identifying a patient at risk. They need to be measured and recorded accurately. The measurements must be taken with sufficient frequency to identify relevant and important changes in physiology, some of which may take place over minutes or even hours. The physiological values must be combined or otherwise transformed to achieve the appropriate score or trigger. This trigger must be meaningful and be able to distinguish between patients who should be seen by the response team from those who do not. The team must arrive in a timely fashion when summoned. Finally the team must be able to make a difference to the outcome of patients. They may be able to do this by initiating treatment, making decisions about admission to critical care areas or by agreeing to limitations on treatment or resuscitation.

Validation of track and trigger scores
Several publications have attempted to validate track and trigger systems. Hodgetts *et al* derived and validated a scoring system [22]. Other studies have examined the ability of subjectively derived systems to identify patients admitted to ICU or who require cardiorespiratory resuscitation or who die [4,11,23,24]. There are limitations in all these studies in the way scores were developed, in the methodology of the studies and analysis of results. However they do provide considerable support for the importance of physiological abnormality and some insights into the measurements likely to be most relevant.

As part of its review of early warning scores ICNARC analysed data provided by British hospitals. Fifteen different track and trigger systems were available for examination. Ten were aggregate scoring systems, one a single parameter system and four combinations. These systems varied with respect to the number and choice of physiological variables, the assignment of scores, trigger thresholds and observed outcomes. Analysis was based upon a composite outcome of death, admission to a critical care unit, 'Do not attempt resuscitation' orders and cardiopulmonary resuscitation. Depending upon hospital, one of these occurred in between 5.7% and 64.7% of patients in the database. The median sensitivities of track and trigger systems were low at 43.3% (interquartile range 25.4 - 69.2%) with median positive predictive values of 36.7% (interquartile range 29.3 - 43.8%). Specificity and negative predictive values were better at 89.5%

(interquartile range 64.2 - 95.7%) and 94.3% (interquartile range 89.5 - 97.0% respectively). Areas under individual receiver operator characteristic (ROC) curves for these systems varied from 0.61 to 0.84. Overall sample sizes were low and their methodologies were imprecise so that firm conclusions cannot be made with any degree of certainty. Furthermore the rapidly changing physiology coupled with infrequent measurement and other practical limitations make it unlikely that these systems could be used to their full potential.

Track and trigger scores are only one part of a system designed to improve the outcome of general ward patients. There are several elements to validating these scores. As has already been shown, there is good evidence showing that abnormal physiology is associated with adverse outcome. Almost all track and trigger scores have been based upon thresholds defined by expert consensus and without evidence to identify the relevant parameters or their values. There is a void between showing that a score can identify appropriate patients and demonstrating that this makes a difference to outcome. This final step is dependent on many things including the training and availability of staff and access to critical care and other resources.

To date the only prospective evaluation of track and trigger systems has taken place in Australia. This study randomised hospitals to having a MET team or continuing without one. After a six month evaluation period, no difference could be detected between the groups with respect to the composite outcome of cardiac arrests, unexpected death, or unplanned ICU admission [15]. However a critical review of the findings suggests that some hospitals performed well even without a MET whereas others did badly despite MET support. Track and trigger systems, MET teams and critical care outreach are all aids to help identify and manage at risk ward patients. If patients are already being managed well, then it will be hard to show an improvement with any intervention. In other hospitals, these initiatives will be beneficial although it is hard to identify what aspect of the system or change of culture is responsible for the benefit. In a few hospitals, systems may be so inefficient or overwhelmed, or the introduction of systems poorly resourced and supported, that change does not take place. Finally it is possible, although unlikely, that early recognition and support for ward patients is of no benefit and their outcome cannot be affected no matter what is done.

Systems are being developed which continuously sample selected physiological values. Preliminary evidence suggests that advanced processing of this data can result in an objectively derived composite score with the ability to identify relevant patients at an earlier stage

[25]. The human brain has a limited ability to retain, process and analyse complex information such as a changing pattern of several streams of physiological recordings. Although subjective assessment (i.e. 'the end of the bed' test) may well be able to detect factors that are not immediately apparent to a machine, advanced analytical methods can synthesise large amounts of continuously collected physiological data. Another advantage is the automation of the system so that certain triggers can initiate warnings through networks, pagers or mobile phones. If such systems can be validated and gain acceptance, there will be no reason why abnormal physiology cannot alert chosen individuals or teams at the earliest opportunity after detectable deterioration occurs.

Conclusions

Many UK hospitals, and an increasing number elsewhere, have introduced some form of physiologically based track and trigger early warning scoring system on general hospital wards. This implies that there is problem identifying and treating groups of sick ward patients and that these systems are seen as one way in which the problem can be addressed. There is good data to show that abnormal physiological values are associated with adverse outcome and there is much sense, as well as precedent, in basing track and trigger systems on these measurements. However improving outcome requires the physiological data to be collected accurately and with sufficient frequency. If a response is triggered, it must be capable of altering outcome in a measurable way. To alter outcome, it is necessary that the response delivers staff with skills, training and experience with the essential equipment, resources and support.

References
1. Knaus WA, Draper EA, Wagner DP, Zimmerman JE. APACHE II: a severity of disease classification system. Critical Care Medicine 1985; 13: 818-29.
2. Le Gall J-R, Lemeshow S, Saulnier F. A new Simplified Acute Physiology Score (SAPS II) based on a European/North American multicenter study. Journal of the American Medical Association 1993; 270: 2957-63.
3. Lemeshow S, Klar J, Teres D *et al.* Mortality probability models for patients in the intensive care unit for 48 or 72 hours: a prospective, multicenter study. Critical Care Medicine 1994; 22: 1351-8.
4. Buist MD, Jarmolowski E, Burton PR, Bernard SA, Waxman BP, Anderson J. Recognising clinical instability in hospital patients before cardiac arrest or unplanned admission to intensive care. A

pilot study in a tertiary-care hospital. Medical Journal of Australia 1999; 171: 22-5.
5. Schein RM, Hazday N, Pena M, Ruben BH, Sprung CL. Clinical antecedents to in-hospital cardiopulmonary arrest. Chest 1990; 98: 1388-92.
6. Kause J, Smith G, Prytherch D, Parr M, Flabouris A, Hillman K. A comparison of antecedents to cardiac arrests, deaths and emergency intensive care admissions in Australia and New Zealand, and the United Kingdom--the ACADEMIA study. Resuscitation 2004; 62: 275-82.
7. Goldhill DR, Worthington L, Mulcahy A, Tarling M. Quality of care before admission to intensive care: Deaths on the wards might be prevented. British Medical Journal 1999; 318: 195.
8. Hillman KM, Bristow PJ, Chey T et al. Antecedents to hospital deaths. Internal Medicine Journal 2001; 31: 343-8.
9. Goldhill DR, White SA, Sumner A. Physiological values and procedures in the 24 hours before ICU admission from the ward. Anaesthesia 1999; 54: 529-34.
10. Cullinane M, Findlay G, Hargraves C, Lucas S. An acute problem. London: National Confidential Enquiry into Patient Outcome and Death, 2005.
11. Goldhill DR, McNarry AF. Physiological abnormalities in early warning scores are related to mortality in adult inpatients. British Journal of Anaesthesia 2004; 92: 882-4.
12. Goldhill DR, McNarry AF, Mandersloot G, McGinley A. A physiologically-based early warning score for ward patients: The association between score and outcome. Anaesthesia 2005; 60: 547-53.
13. Goldhill DR, McNarry AF, Hadjianastassiou VG, Tekkis PP. The longer patients are in hospital before intensive care admission the higher their mortality. Intensive Care Medicine 2004; 30: 1908-13.
14. McBride J, Knight D, Piper J, Smith GB. Long-term effect of introducing an early warning score on respiratory rate charting on general wards. Resuscitation 2005; 65: 41-4.
15. Hillman K, Chen J, Cretikos M et al. Introduction of the medical emergency team (MET) system: a cluster-randomised controlled trial. Lancet 2005; 365: 2091-7.
16. Nurmi J, Harjola VP, Nolan J, Castren M. Observations and warning signs prior to cardiac arrest. Should a medical emergency team intervene earlier? Acta Anaesthesiologica Scandinavica 2005; 49: 702-6.
17. Jones D, Bates S, Warrillow S et al. Circadian pattern of activation of the medical emergency team in a teaching hospital. Critical Care 2005; 9: R303-R306.

18. Lee A, Bishop G, Hillman KM, Daffurn K. The Medical Emergency Team. Anaesthesia & Intensive Care 1995; 23: 183-6.
19. Morgan RJM, Williams F, Wright MM. An early warning score for the early detection of patients with impending illness. Clinical Intensive Care 8, 100. 1997.
20. Department of Health and Modernsation Agency. The National Outreach Report 2003. London: Department of Health. 2003..
21. Gao H, McDonnell A, Harrison DA, *et al.* Systematic review and evaluation of physiological track and trigger warning systems for identifying at-risk patients on the ward. Intensive Care Medicine 2007; 33: 667-679.
22. Hodgetts TJ, Kenward G, Vlachonikolis IG, Payne S, Castle N. The identification of risk factors for cardiac arrest and formulation of activation criteria to alert a medical emergency team. Resuscitation 2002; 54: 125-31.
23. Goldhill DR, Worthington L, Mulcahy A, Tarling M, Sumner A. The patient at risk team: Identifying and managing seriously ill ward patients. Anaesthesia 1999; 54: 853-60.
24. Subbe CP, Kruger M, Rutherford P, Gemmel L. Validation of a modified early warning score in medical admissions. Quarterly Journal of Medicine 2001; 94: 521-6.
25. Goldhill DR. Of missiles and medicine: early warning systems. Anaesthesia 2006; 61: 209-11.
26. Buist MD, Moore GE, Bernard SA, Waxman BP, Anderson JN, Nguyen TV. Effects of a medical emergency team on reduction of incidence of and mortality from unexpected cardiac arrests in hospital: preliminary study. British Medical Journal 2002; 324: 387-390.

3: Myocardial ischaemia; when to intervene

DR ROBERT SAPSFORD

Introduction
Almost 30% of general intensive care unit (ICU) patients have previously documented ischaemic heart disease (IHD) and in one series 14% of patrients had evidence of prior left ventricular dysfunction [1]. In addition many post-operative admissions to critical care are precipitated by peri-operative cardiac events, which despite pre-operative risk stratification and secondary prevention treatments still cause significant morbidity (18%) and mortality (3.4%) in patients undergoing vascular surgery [2]. Therefore it is no surprise that myocardial ischaemia is encountered commonly in critically ill patients, with evidence of cardiac events in 10 - 35% of patients [3, 4]. In this chapter, the interpretation of cardiac biomarkers (troponins) and the recent developments in the management of acute coronary syndromes will be discussed with reference to critically ill patients.

Identification
The prevalence of myocardial ischaemia depends upon the detection techniques. Looking for ischaemia with the electrocardiogram (ECG) in the ICU is limited by the use of multiple drugs, posture and respiration and so may miss up to 80% of ischaemic episodes [5]. Transient ST depression (> 1 mm lasting over 1 min) were detected in eight of 76 consecutive patients admitted to ICU for non-cardiac conditions. In these eight patients, a total of 37 ischaemic events were seen of which 96% were clinically silent, despite transient ischaemia being predictive of cardiac complications [6]. Whilst prolonged ST depression lasting longer than 60 min is 95% specific and has a reasonable positive predictive value (80%) for identifying patients who will have a raised cardiac biomarkers, it lacks sensitivity (31%) [7]. However, despite the ECG's poor sensitivity it may suggest the presence of more functionally significant epicardial lesions than biomarkers alone, thereby identifying patients who may benefit from coronary revascularisation.

Clinically recognised cardiac dysfunction (as defined as myocardial infarction, unstable angina, cardiac arrest or congestive heart failure) was found in 21% of ICU patients and may be a better predictor of outcome than troponin levels alone [8]. Also in patients admitted with acute coronary syndromes who required prolonged critical care for multiple organ dysfunction, the main independent predictor for mortality was the severity of heart failure and presence of co-morbidities [9, 10]. This may also explain why patients with higher heart rates (> 95 beats/min for > 12 hours) are at increased risk of adverse cardiac events [11].

Troponins

Studies identifying cardiac injury have been undertaken since the introduction of cardiac troponins as they are a specific and sensitive marker of myocyte necrosis. In patients presenting with ischaemic chest pain, troponins have proved to be valuable prognostic indicators. Two cardiac troponins, T and I, are used in the diagnosis of acute coronary syndromes. The latter has several assays each with differing reference ranges and therefore it is important when interpreting results to be aware of the assay used.

In a prospective study of 209 ICU patients, 32 (15%) were found to have elevated cardiac troponins but only four patients displayed clinical signs and symptoms. The mortality in the troponin positive group was significantly higher (42%) compared to those who were troponin negative (15%). There were also differences in mechanical ventilation (66% versus 27%), hypotension (75% versus 50%) and longer ICU stays (5.3 versus 3.1 days) [12].

However, it is now recognised that troponins can also be elevated in patients without acute coronary syndrome, particularly in sepsis and multiple organ failure. Such elevations are still associated with an adverse prognosis. Wu *et al* [13] found troponin rises in 49 of 108 (45%) critically ill patients without known acute coronary syndrome or cardiac disease. Those patients with elevated levels had a greater incidence of multi-organ failure and mortality.

Minkin *et al* [14] retrospectively reviewed patients admitted to a medical ICU during a six month period and found 41 of the 132 patients (31%) were troponin I positive and had a hospital mortality of 39%. However, the statistical association of mortality with positive troponin levels was weak for early mortality and non-existent for long-term mortality suggesting it may be of limited value if used to screen all patients. These results conflicted with a prospective study in which 217 consecutive patients over a 6 month study period were assessed using troponin I as a measure of myocardial injury. Troponin elevation was found in 70 (32%) patients; mortality within this group was 51% compared with only 16% in the troponin negative group. This suggests that a positive troponin rise could identify patients at increased risk of death [15].

In high risk ICU patients as judged by a history of coronary artery disease or at least two other risk factors (including age >65 years, Q waves on ECG, diabetes, hypertension, hyperlipidaemia, smoking and chronic renal failure), a positive troponin rise was found in 38 of 101 patients (38%) [16]. Only four of episodes of myocardial ischaemia were suspected clinically and only 14 (36%) of troponin positive patients had ischaemic ECG changes on holter monitoring. Predictors of a troponin rise were prolonged ischaemia (> 60 min of ST depression), high APACHE II score and norepinephrine use. Elevated troponin was associated with increased both early and late mortality [16].

In a rigorous study, 58 consecutive patients admitted to an ICU for reasons other than suspected acute coronary syndrome were assessed by biomarkers, ejection fraction and 30-day mortality. Thirty-four patients (55%) were troponin positive and also suffered a significantly higher mortality (22.4% versus 5.2%) and lower ejection fractions compared to the troponin negative cohort. Inflammatory mediators (tumour necrosis factor (TNF)-alpha and interleukin (IL)-6 levels) were increased in the troponin positive patients. Interestingly, flow limiting coronary artery disease was not present at autopsy nor suggested by stress-echocardiograph in 72% of the troponin positive group [17]. This suggests that a detectable troponin level was not necessarily linked to significant epicardial stenosis which would be likely to benefit from coronary intervention and so troponin levels should not be used for screening in isolation.

Pathophysiology of plaque rupture
An important consideration in acute coronary syndrome management is that previously asymptomatic plaques causing narrowing but not functional flow limitation frequently rupture. Atherosclerotic plaques are extremely common and up to 85% of the population above 50 years of age may have significant intimal thickening [18]. Intravascular ultrasound techniques and histopathological examination demonstrate that plaque structure varies with respect to the thickness of the covering fibrous plaque and number of inflammatory cells present at the plaque margins. It is the degradation of the collagen surface together with the shear stresses imposed on the plaque which seem to promote rupture and the subsequent cascade of thrombosis and repair.

When plaque rupture occurs, progression to complete or partial thrombotic vessel occlusion is dependent on a delicate balance between thrombosis and endogenous thrombolysis (mediated by plasminogen activator inhibitor-1 (PAI-1) and prostacyclin). Flow

MYOCARDIAL ISCHAEMIA; WHEN TO INTERVENE

characteristics in the vessel (low flows promoting thrombus generation), smaller vessel size and increased coagulation factors levels (e.g. in sepsis or after surgery) promote thrombosis. Therefore, critically ill patients have a tendency towards thrombosis and any unstable plaques which in other circumstances may have been repaired uneventfully may partially or fully occlude the vessel and so initiate troponin release.

Figure 1. Myocardial definition, myocyte damage and relationship to biochemical markers. (ACC: American College of Cardiology, WHO: World Health Organisation, BCS: British Cardiac Society, UA: Unstable Angina, MI: Myocardial Infarction, ULN: Upper limit of Normal)
Joint European Society / ACC criteria for acute, evolving or recent MI – one of following:
   1) Pathological findings of acute MI
   2) Typical rise and fall of biomarker of myocardial necrosis with at least 1 of following:
        a. Ischaemic symptoms
        b. Q waves
        c. Ischaemic ECG changes
        d. Coronary artery intervention

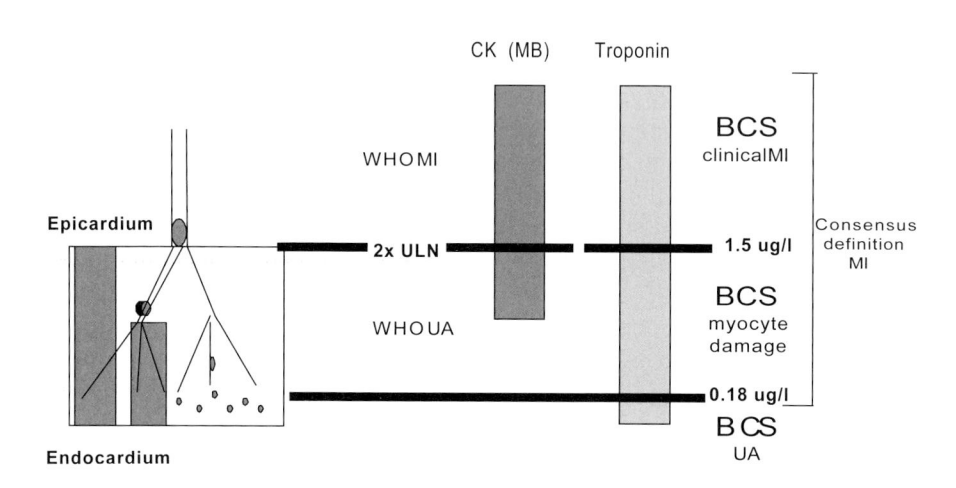

However, any cause of myocyte damage will cause troponin release such as embolisation or direct toxic effects on the myocardium (e.g. chemotherapy, viral agents or inotropes) [19]. Therefore whilst troponins are specific for myocyte damage, they are not always indicative of epicardial coronary disease. This has important implications when deciding on the optimal management strategies as only a proportion of patients will benefit from conventional acute coronary syndrome revascularisation treatments.

Nomenclature of acute coronary syndrome
To deal with this uncertainty the British Cardiac Society (BCS) proposed diagnostic categories which will improve consistency in diagnosing myocardial infarctions (Figure 1). In troponin negative patients, it is important to realise that whilst myocyte damage has not occurred, this does not exclude the presence of significant epicardial stenoses, with left main stem or three vessel coronary disease being found in 20% of troponin negative patients. The diagnostic criteria also include the presenting ECG and symptoms which may not always be available in ICU [20].

In acute coronary syndrome, lower levels of troponin release predict possible further complications and subsequent mortality rather than the immediate risk imposed by the full thickness epicardial artery occlusions. Under these circumstances, the risk of arrhythmias is high; 60% of all deaths in this group have occurred before hospital admission and subsequent mortality is determined by left ventricular systolic dysfunction (Table 1).

Table 1. Acute Coronary Syndromes (ACS) – proposed nomenclature and relationship to mortality (adapted from the BCS working group paper [20]).

	ACS with unstable angina	ACS with myocyte necrosis	ACS with clinical myocardial infarction
Marker	Troponin undectable	Troponin below MI threshold	Troponin above MI threshold
ECG	Normal ST and T waves or transient changes		Persistent ST and T wave changes (may evolve into Q waves
LV function	No measurable dysfunction	→	Systolic Dysfunction

Management of acute coronary syndromes

The first decision is whether the ECG changes or biomarker rise represents an acute coronary syndrome related to epicardial vessel disease. Additional information from echocardiography, biomarker profiles and ECG progression may be helpful. On occasions radionuclear scans or magnetic resonance imaging (MRI) may be used but logistics restrict application in the critically ill.

An acute coronary syndrome is suspected if the ECG shows ST elevation or the development of new left bundle branch block (LBBB); under these circumstances, emergency reperfusion therapies should be applied. Patients presenting with ECGs fulfilling the criteria for thrombolysis or percutaneous revascularisation are a minority (only 9% of cases present with ST segment elevation). Even for patients discharged with a final diagnosis of myocardial infarction, only 44% were eligible for thrombolysis [21]. Thrombolytic agents increase degradation of established thrombus and include streptokinase, tissue plasminogen activator (tPA) and newer agents such as tenecteplase (TNK). Newer agents have increased efficacy but are dependent on time following onset of symptoms to have optimal effect. Even so they may only re-establish patency in 50 – 65% of patients when assessed by angiography at 90 minutes following treatment [22].

The patient should be regularly assessed and monitored for acute arrhythmias and haemodynamic complications. They also require supplementary oxygen, analgesia and anti-platelet agents. Following reperfusion with thrombolytic agents only 60-70% achieve target vessel patency even with the latest agents. This is important as artery patency is prognostic; the mortality for failed reperfusion is 12% compared with 4% for patent arteries [23]. The routine use of salvage percutaneous revascularisation to open arteries of patients with clinical evidence of failed reperfusion following thrombolysis has not demonstrated any overall benefit despite increasing coronary artery patency from 65% to 87% [24]. Appropriate secondary prevention therapies such as beta-blockers, statins, angiotensin converting enzyme inhibitors, aspirin and clopidogrel should be started as early as possible.

In acute coronary syndrome with no immediate indications for thrombolysis on the initial ECG, repeated ECGs and risk assessment are used to target appropriate therapies. A variety of risk stratifying scores exist of which the TIMI risk [25] and GRACE scores [26] are frequently used and may identify higher risk cohorts for earlier treatment with more aggressive agents such as glycoprotein IIb/IIIa antagonists.

Anti-thrombotic medical treatments
Treatment is directed principally against the underlying mechanisms precipitating ischaemia. In the case of acute coronary syndromes preventing further platelet deposition, restoring flow in occluded arteries and reducing myocardial oxygen demand are all treatment aims.

Platelet deposition is the first element of thrombus formation. Loading doses of aspirin and / or clopidogrel can be used for rapid effect. Aspirin affects the arachadonic acid pathway within the platelets and vessel wall and reduces thromboxane mediated platelet aggregation; it may also inhibit prothrombin. Clopidogrel is an adenosine diphosphate antagonist which binds irreversibly to the platelets inhibiting adenosine diphosphate mediated aggregation. In combination with aspirin it produces a synergistic effect and is used with aspirin in higher risk acute coronary syndrome [27] and following stenting. It can be used alone in cases of aspirin intolerance but has not been shown to offer any additional reduction in gastrointestinal bleeds. The combination of aspirin and clopidogrel is associated with an increased bleeding risk; six significant bleeds occur for every 1000 patients treated with the combination therapy. However, the rate of stent thrombosis for patients not treated with either agent is around 10% [28].

Heparin can also reduce thrombus formation. Intravenous heparin has a short half life and so is suitable for patients at increased bleeding risk. However it may have a variable therapeutic effect as monitored by the activated partial thromboplastin time (APTT). This led to the development of more specific and stable low molecular weight heparins (LMWH) and studies have shown benefit in acute coronary syndromes [29]. They have to be used with caution in renal failure due to their renal excretion and should be used at half dose if the estimated creatinine clearance is below 30 ml/min.

Glycoprotein IIb/IIIa antagonists are extremely effective anti-platelet agents which exert their effect via the IIb/IIIa receptors, the most numerous receptors on platelets. The current agents whether small molecules (eptifibatide / tirofiban) or antibodies (abciximab) have to be given intravenously as a bolus followed by 12-18 hours infusion before and after percutaneous revascularisation. They carry similar bleeding risks and contra-indications to thrombolytic agents. They reduce peri-procedural myocardial events particularly in the higher risk patients, resulting in a 30-40% reduction in mortality, myocardial infarction or urgent target vessel revascularisation [30]. The use of these agents prior to revascularisation in patients treated with medical therapy alone has not been shown to be of benefit [31].

Anti-ischaemic and secondary prevention treatments
Reduction of myocardial oxygen demand is achieved by reducing heart rate and afterload and in coronary care is best achieved using beta-blockade. However, therapeutic beta-blockade may be relatively contra-indicated in many ICU patients who typically require inotropic support. Nitrates are helpful for relieving ischaemic pain and pre-load but have not been shown to alter progression of myocyte damage or subsequent mortality [32].

Statins are now widely used in atheromatous disease. The MIRACL study [33] demonstrated benefit with the early administration of high dose statin (i.e. atorvastatin 80 mg) which reduced the number of hospital admissions within 6 weeks suggesting an extra effect to those achieved by simple cholesterol reduction. This 'pleiotropic effect' may be mediated through a reduced inflammatory response and so may imply that it would be preferable not to withdraw statins in the acute phase unless their continued use was contra-indicated because of concomitant renal, muscular or hepatic dysfunction.

Angiotensin converting enzyme inhibitors and possibly angiotensin receptor antagonists appear to reduce subsequent vascular events to a greater extent than would be expected by the protective effect of lowering blood pressure alone. Angiotensin converting enzyme inhibitors reduce afterload, left ventricular end diastolic pressure and thereby the degree of atrial stretch; the incidence of atrial arrhythmias is also reduced [34]. They are of proven value in left ventricular systolic dysfunction reducing mortality and morbidity and should be started when the patient is haemodynamically stable.

Other anti-anginal agents include nicorandil which is a potassium channel agonist and has additional nitrate-like actions; it has protective effects in patients with ischaemic chest pain [35]. The calcium channel antagonists diltiazem and verapamil whilst suitable for preventing ischaemic chest pain and providing rate reduction should be avoided in patients with reduced left ventricular systolic function. The role of the latest anti-anginal agent ivabradine which slows the sinus node rate via action on the 'funny' (f) channels has not been tested outside patients with stable angina.

Percutaneous Revascularisation

Percutaneous intervention (PCI) is a rapidly expanding field which enables the visualisation of the coronary lumen and insertion of an expandable balloon (angioplasty) or more commonly a balloon and stent (an expandable metal lattice) resulting in compression and outward radial displacement of the atheromatous plaque. The technology is rapidly developing and stents are now used in over 80% procedures and have been shown to reduce re-stenosis by 30% and the need for target vessel revascularisation by 30% at six months [36]. Further developments in both stent design and the use of drug eluting stents which limit endothelialisation and thereby reducing re-stenosis have seen re-stenosis rates reduce to < 1% at six months [37]. Their disadvantage is the need for more prolonged anti-platelet regimens for a minimum of 1 year which may influence the timing of elective surgery and potentially increase the risk should the anti-platelet regime be interrupted.

If the anti-platelet regime is stopped or co-morbidities lead to low flow rates or sepsis following stent insertion, the greatest risk is sub-acute stent thrombosis. This has the potential complications of death (20%) and myocardial infarction (40%). Sub-acute stent thrombosis appears to be one reason why operative procedures carried out early after stenting do not reduce peri-operative risks but may actually increase them [38]. In cases where surgery is urgent and the bleeding risk precludes the continued use of anti-platelet agents, the risk of per-operative stent thrombosis may approach 5-10% [28].

The complications of percutaneous revascularisation vary between 1-10% depending on the circumstances. Percutaneous revascularisation and stenting can be thought of as providing a controlled plaque rupture in the presence of potent anti-platelet agents to prevent occlusive thrombus formation. Nevertheless distal embolisation and abrupt vessel occlusion (particularly of side branches in complex lesions) do result in significant troponin rises and the long-term significance of these low level troponin releases remains controversial.

Vascular complications occur in 1-5% of cases particularly with anticoagulation or following thrombolysis. These can vary from localised haematoma, pseudoanuerysm, arterio-venous fistula to retroperitoneal haemorrhage. Transfusions is needed in 1% of patients [39]

Contrast induced nephropathy (CIN) is particularly relevant to the critically ill patients who often have a degree of renal impairment or concomitant use of other nephrotoxic agents. The use of large quantities of contrast during cardiac procedures may lead to contrast induced nephropathy with increased creatinine levels after 48 hours; this can progress to acute tubular necrosis. Risk factors for contrast induced nephropathy include prior renal dysfunction, diabetics, older age and a pre-renal component [40]. The dangers can be reduced with fluid hydration before and after the procedure and stopping other nephrotoxic agents. Intravenous N-acetylcysteine has recently been shown to have a positive effect both on the reduction of contrast induced nephropathy and an improvement in mortality when given during primary angioplasty [41].

Cardiogenic shock
Around 5 to 10% of patients with myocardial infarction will develop cardiogenic shock with a 30-day mortality approaching 90%. The definition of cardiogenic shock includes hypotension (systemic arterial blood pressure < 90 mmHg) with evidence of hypoperfusion (cardiac index < 2 l/min/m^2) and pulmonary congestion (mean pulmonary wedge pressure > 20 mmHg). Although trials in this area have only enrolled small numbers of patients, they do suggest a significant reduction in mortality at 30 days from 58% in the non-revascularised group to 21% in those treated with early revascularisation including circulatory support with intra-aortic balloon counterpulsation [42]. A later trial supported this with a reduced mortality (45%) in the revascularised group compared to solely supportive therapies (including intra-aortic balloon pump with a mortality of 88%) [43].

In a recent review the mortality from cardiogenic shock in patients treated conservatively showed that mortality remained unchanged even with the use of thrombolytic agents suggesting that primary angioplasty may be the treatment of choice. Certainly the high procedural success rates (> 75%) and lower mortality has led to percutaneous revascularisation becoming the treatment of choice in acute coronary syndrome complicated by cardiogenic shock. Whilst coronary artery bypass grafting may be expected to offer similar benefits, the logistics of urgent access to this form of revascularisation suggest that percutaneous revascularisation would offer the optimal form of revascularisation [44].

The use of intra-aortic balloon counterpulsation is increasing both for pre-optimisation for coronary artery bypass grafting especially in patients at high risk identified as redo coronary artery bypass grafting, unstable angina, left main stem stenosis, reduced ejection fraction (defined as an ejection fraction < 30%) and diffuse coronary disease

[45]. Their use reduces post-operative mortality and morbidity, shortens ICU stays and reduces drug consumption. Such adjuvant therapy is becoming more widespread in high risk percutaneous revascularisation patients especially for left main stem stenting and patients with cardiogenic shock.

Conclusion
Manifestations of cardiac ischaemia should considered and actively sought in the critical ill patient especially as ST segment shifts though specific are unreliable and troponins sensitive but lack specificity for epicardial coronary disease. Elevation of cardiac troponins should prompt a re-assessment of the patient with consideration for the use of further non-invasive assessments (ECGs and echocardiography) which may give information as to the underlying cause, degree of left ventricular dysfunction and suggest the need for more urgent revascularisation (Figure 2).

Lowering the myocardial oxygen demand with heart rate suppression to promote longer diastolic filling times and afterload reduction with beta-blockade would be optimal but is frequently prevented by co-existent pathology and the need for inotropic support. Reduction of blood pressure and pre-load with nitrates or more potent vasodilators can be considered especially in the setting of hypertensive pulmonary oedema.

Preventing or limiting the thrombotic tendency with anti-platelet agents and anticoagulants will reduce the chances of further cardiac events. Where ischaemia remains refractory or cardiogenic shock ensues percutaneous revascularisation should be considered. Knowledge of the potential complications and limitations imposed if aggressive anti-platelet therapies can not be used will help inform this decision.

MYOCARDIAL ISCHAEMIA; WHEN TO INTERVENE

Figure 2. Suggested algorithm for assessment of suspected cardiac ischaemia in critical care patients. Shaded boxes: Consider revascularisation if present. (IHD: Ischaemic heart disease, LVD: Left ventricle dysfunction, LBBB: Left bundle branch block, ASC: Acute coronary syndrome, PCI: Percutaneous intervention, CAVG: Coronary artery vein graft)

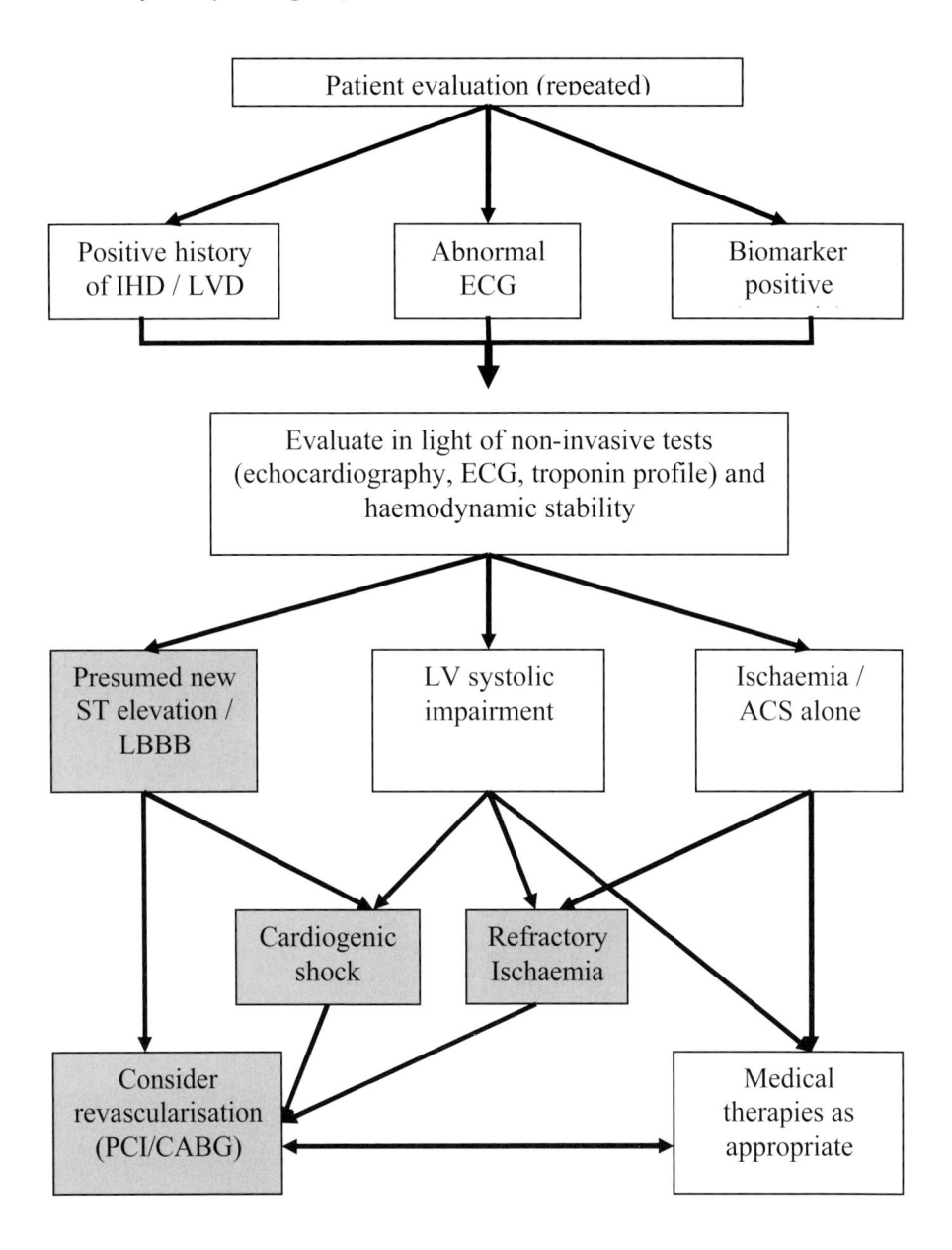

References

1. Walsh TS, McClelland DB, Lee RJ, et al. Prevalence of ischaemic heart disease at admission to intensive care and its influence on red cell transfusion thresholds: multi-centre Scottish Study. British Journal of Anaesthesia 2005; 94: 445-452.
2. Mackey WC, Fleisher LA, Haider S, et al. Peri-operative myocardial ischaemic injury in high risk vascular surgery patients: incidence and clinical significance in a prospective clinical trial. Journal of Vascular Surgery 2006; 43: 533-538.
3. Hurford WE, Favorito F. Association of myocardial ischaemia with failure to wean from mechanical ventilation. Critical Care Medicine 1995; 23: 1475-1480.
4. Srivastava S, Chatila W, Amoateng-Adjepong Y, et al. Myocardial ischaemia and weaning failure in patients with coronary artery disease: and update. Critical Care Medicine 1999 27: 2109-2112.
5. Biaginin A, L'Abbate A, Testa R, et al. Unreliability of conventional visual electrocardiographic monitoring for detection of transient ST segment changes in a coronary care unit. European Heart Journal 1984; 5: 784-791.
6. Booker KJ, Holm K, Drew BJ, et al. Frequency and outcomes of transient myocardial ischaemia in critically ill adults admitted for non-cardiac conditions. American Journal of Critical Care 2003; 12: 508-516.
7. Landesburg G, Vesselov Y, Einav S, Goodman S, Sprung CL, Weissman C. Myocardial Ischaemia, cardiac troponin and long-term survival of high cardiac risk critically ill intensive care unit patients. Critical Care Medicine 2005; 33: 1439-1441.
8. Kollef MH, Landeson JH, Eisenberg PR. Clinically recognized cardiac dysfunction; an independent determinant of mortality among critically ill patients. Is there a role for serial measurement of cardiac troponin I? Chest 1997; 111: 1340-1347.
9. Zahger D, Maimon N, Novack V, et al. Clinical characteristics and prognostic factors in patients with complicated acute coronary syndromes requiring prolonged mechanical ventilation. American Journal of Cardiology 2005; 96: 1644-1648.
10. Lesage A, Ramakers M, Daubin C, et al. Complicated acute myocardial infarction requiring mechanical ventilation in the intensive care unit: prognostic factors of clinical outcome in a series of 157 patients. Critical Care Medicine 2004; 32: 100-105.
11. Sander O, Welters ID, Foex P, Sear JW. Impact of elevated heart rate on incidence of major cardiac events in critically ill patients with a high risk of cardiac complications. Critical Care Medicine 2005; 33: 81-88.

12. Guest TM, Ramanathan AV, Tuteur PG, Schechtman KB, Landenson JH, Jaffe AS. Myocardial injury in critically ill patients. A frequent unrecognised complication. Journal of the American Medical Association 1995; 273: 1945-1954.
13. Wu TT, Yuan A, Chen CY, et al. Cardiac troponin I levels are a risk factor for mortality and multiple organ failure in non-cardiac critically ill patients and have an additive effect to the APACHE II score in outcome prediction. Shock 2004; 22: 95-101.
14. Minkin R, Cotiga D, Noack S, Dobrescu A, Homel P, Shapiro JM. Use of admission troponin in critically ill medical patients. Journal of Intensive Care Medicine 2005; 20: 332-338.
15. Quenot JP, Le Teuff G, Quantin C, et al. Myocardial injury in critically ill patients: relation to increased cardiac troponin I and hospital mortality. Chest 2005; 128: 2758-2764.
16. Landesberg C, Vesselov Y, Einav S, Goodman S, Sprung CL, Weissman C. Myocardial ischaemia, cardiac troponin and long-term survival of high cardiac risk critically ill intensive care unit patients. Critical Care Medicine 2005; 33: 1281-1287.
17. Ammann P, Maggiorini M, Bertel O, et al. Troponin as a risk factor for mortality in critically ill patients without acute coronary syndrome. Journal of the American College of Cardiologists 2003; 41: 2004-2009.
18. Tuzcu EM, Kapadia S, Tutar E, et al. High prevalence of coronary atherosclerosis in asymptomatic teenagers and young adults: evidence from intravascular ultrasound. Circulation 2001; 103: 2705-2710.
19. Ammann P, Pfisterer M, Fehr T, Rickli H. Raised cardiac troponins. British Medical Journal 2005; 328: 1028-1029.
20. Fox KAA, Birkhead J, Wilcox R, Knight C, Barth J. British Cardiac Society Working Group on the definition of myocardial infarction. Heart 2004; 90: 603-609.
21. French JK, Williams BF, Hart HH, et al. Prospective evaluation of eligibility for thrombolytic therapy in acute myocardial infarction. British Medical Journal 1996; 312: 1637-1641.
22. Cannon CP, McCabe CH, Diver DJ on behalf of the TIMI -4 (Thrombolysis in Myocardial Infarction -4) Study Group. Comparison of front loaded recombinant tissue type plasminogen activator, anistreplase, and combination thrombolytic therapy for acute myocardial infarction: results of the Thrombolysis in Myocardial Infarction (TIMI) 4 trial. Journal of the American College of Cardiologists 1994; 24: 1602-1610.
23. Ohman E, Califf RM, Topol EJ, et al. Consequences of re-occlusion after successful reperfusion therapy in acute myocardial infarction. Thrombolysis in Acute Myocardial Infarction (TAMI) study group. Circulation 1990; 82: 781-791.

24. Gibson CM, Cannon CP, Greene RM *et al* on behalf of the TIMI - 4 (Thrombolysis in Myocardial Infarction -4) Study Group. Rescue angioplasty in the thrombolysis in myocardial infarction – (TIMI) 4 trial. American Journal of Cardiology 1997; 8: 21-26.
25. Sabatine MS, Antman EM. The thrombolysis in myocardial infarction risk score in unstable angina/non-ST-segment elevation myocardial infarction. Journal of the American College of Cardiologists 2003; 41: 89S-95S.
26. Eagle KA, Lim MJ, Budaj A, *et al* on behalf of the GRACE Investigators. A robust prediction model for all forms of acute coronary syndromes: estimating the risk of in-hospital death and myocardial infarction in the Global Registry of Acute Coronary Events Registry. Journal of the American College of Cardiologists 2003; 41: 353A.
27. Yusuf S, Zhao F, Mehta SR, Chrolavicius S, Tognoni G, Fox KK; Clopidogrel in Unstable Angina to Prevent Recurrent Events Trial Investigators. Effects of clopidogrel in addition to aspirin in patients with acute coronary syndromes without ST segment elevation. New England Journal of Medicine 2001; 345: 494-502.
28. Schatz RA, Baim DS, Leon M, *et al*. Clinical experience with the Palmer-Schatz coronary stent: initial results of a multi-centre study. Circulation 1991; 83: 148-161.
29. FRISC Investigators. Fragmin and fast revascularisation during instability in coronary artery disease II Investigators. Long-term low-molecular-mass heparin in unstable coronary disease: FRISC II prospective randomized multi-center study. Lancet 1999; 354: 701-707.
30. Department of Cardiology. Platelet glycoprotein IIb/IIIa receptor blockade and low dose heparin during percutaneous coronary revascularisation: the EPILOG investigators. New England Journal of Medicine 1997; 336: 1689-1696.
31. Simoons ML; The GUSTO-IV-ACS Investigators. Global utilization of strategies to open occluded coronary arteries – IV – acute coronary syndromes. Effect of glycoprotein IIb/IIIa receptor blocker abciximab on outcome in patients with acute coronary syndromes without early coronary revascularisation: the GUSTO-IV-ACS randomized trial. Lancet 2001; 357: 1915-1924.
32. ISIS- study group. ISIS-4: a randomised factorial trial assessing early oral captopril, oral mononitrate, and intravenous magnesium sulphate in 58,050 patients with suspected acute myocardial infarction. Lancet 1995; 345: 669-685.
33. Scwartz GG, Olsson AG, Ezekowitz MD, *et al* and the Myocardial Ischemia Reduction with Aggressive Cholesterol Lowering (MIRACL) Study Investigators. Effects of atorvastatin on early recurrent ischaemic events in acute coronary syndromes.

The Myocardial Ischaemia Reduction with Aggressive Cholesterol Lowering (MIRACL) study: a randomized controlled trial. Journal of the American Medical Association 2001; 285: 1711-1718.
34. Dahlof B, Devereux RB, Kjeldson S, *et al* and the LIFE Study Group. Cardiovascular morbidity and mortality in the Losartan Intervention For Endpoint reduction in hypertension study (LIFE): a randomized trial against atenolol. Lancet 2002; 359: 995-1003.
35. The IONA Study Group. Effect of nicorandil on coronary events in patients with stable angina: the Impact of Nicorandil in Angina (IONA) randomized trial. Lancet 2002; 359: 1269-1275.
36. Fischman D, Leon MB, Baim DS, *et al*. A randomised comparison of coronary artery stent placement and balloon angioplasty in the treatment of coronary artery disease. New England Journal of Medicine 1994; 331: 496-501.
37. Morice M-C, Serruys PW, Sousa JE, *et al*. A randomised comparison of a sirolimus-eluting stent with a standard stent for coronary revascularisation. New England Journal of Medicine 2002; 346: 1173-1180.
38. Cutlip DE, Baim DS, Ho KKL, *et al*. Stent thrombosis in the modern era: a pooled analysis of multi-centre coronary stent clinical trials. Circulation 2001; 103: 1967-1971.
39. Nasser TK, Mohler ER, Wilensky RL, Hathaway DR. Peripheral vascular complications following coronary interventional procedures. Clinical Cardiology 1995; 18: 609-614.
40. McCullough PA, Wolyn R, Rocher LL, Levin RN, O'Neill WW. Acute renal failure after coronary intervention: incidence, risk factors, and relationship to mortality. American Medical Journal 1997; 103: 368-375.
41. Marenzi G, Assanelli E, Marana I, *et al*. N-acetylcysteine and contrast induced nephropathy in primary angioplasty. New England Journal of Medicine 2006; 354: 2773-2782.
42. Lindholme MG, Aldershvile J, Sungreen C, Jorgensen E, Saunamaki K, Boesgaard S. The effect of early revascularization in cardiogenic shock complicating acute myocardial infarction. A single centre experience. European Journal of Heart Failure 2003; 5: 73-79.
43. Hochman JS, Sleeper LA, Webb JG, *et al*. Early revascularisation in acute myocardial infarction complicated by cardiogenic shock. SHOCK Investigators. Should we Emergently Revascularise Occluded Coronaries For Cardiogenic Shock. New England Journal of Medicine 1999; 341: 625-634.
44. Chou TM, Amidon TM, Ports TA, Wolfe CL. Cardiogenic shock: thrombolysis or angioplasty? Journal of Intensive Care Medicine 1996; 11: 37-48.

45. Christenson JT, Schmuziger M, Simonet F. Effective surgical management of high-risk coronary patients using preoperative intra-aortic balloon counterpulsation therapy. Cardiovascular Surgery 2001; 9: 383-390.

4: Echocardiography in the Intensive Care Unit

DR SEAN BENNETT

Introduction
Ultrasound is the latest tool to be widely introduced into intensive care units (ICUs). Part of this development is echocardiography and the evaluation of cardiac function in the critically ill patient. Many reviews and editorials were written on this in the late 1990s [1-3]. All describe the various applications of ultrasound and echocardiography. However, it is uncommon to find ultrasound as the primary tool in patient management because machines are still expensive despite being cheaper than a decade ago. Expertise is required to gain good information and continued practice to maintain skills. Ultrasound also gives the operator both monitoring and diagnostic information and some anaesthetists may not comfortable with the latter. Finally, the technique can only give intermittent information that will depend on the presence of a skilled operator.

Types of ultrasound machine
Until recently, vascular, thoracic and abdominal ultrasound each required a different machine. Now modern machines are capable of scanning most sites with the operator simply changing probes. This includes transoesophageal echocardiograhpy (TOE). The probes have their own frequency bands which even portable machines can process. This has reduced the cost and improved the availability of information. Scanning central veins has been largely accepted but scanning for pleural effusions is as easy (Figures 1 & 2). However other scans such as estimating renal artery blood flow may be difficult and require constant practice to avoid errors.

Transthoracic versus transoesophageal echocardiography
Transthoracic echocardiography (TTE) is dependent upon the quality of the acoustic window. Various studies suggest that good views are obtainable in only a minority of critical care patients. Optimal views are found in only 25% of patients, sub-optimal in 70% and the heart may not be seen in 6% [4]. However intensivists have found that although the window may not be perfect, the information they require can be obtained in up to 97% of patients [5]. Ventilated lung, dressings and drains mean that many views will be impossible to obtain. Still the non-invasive nature of transthoracic echocardiography, the use of tissue harmonics (in which harmonics

CRITICAL CARE FOCUS 14: UPDATES

Figure 1. A large left pleural effusion in the centre of the image with lung on the right.

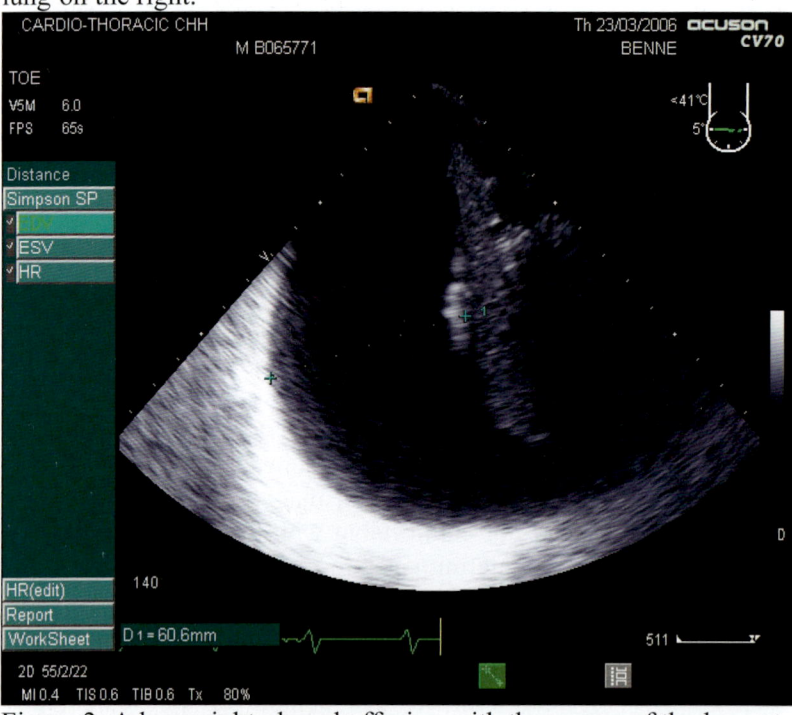

Figure 2. A large right pleural effusion with the corner of the lung at the apex.

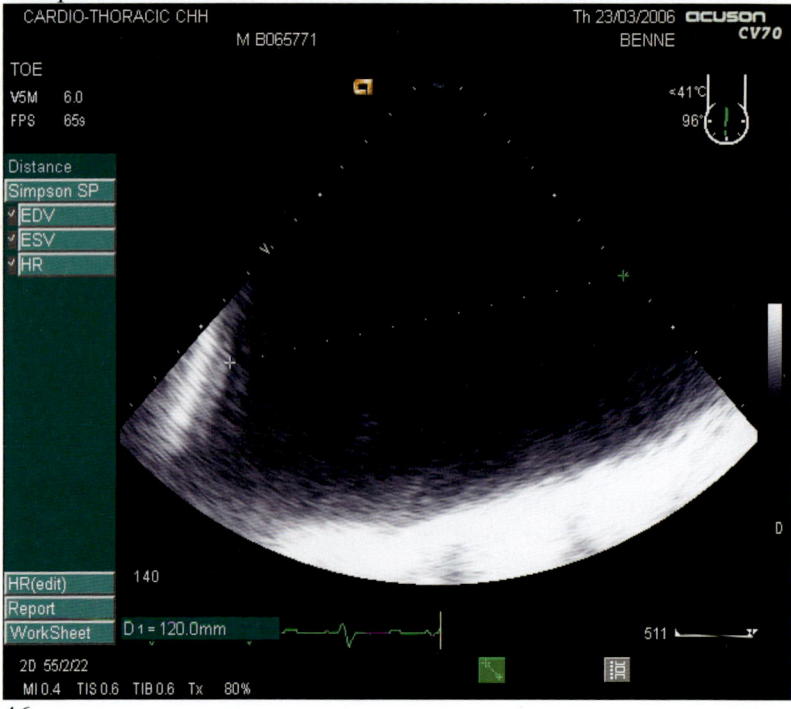

generated by the passage of sound through tissue are selectively dampened or amplified to enhance the image) and the goal directed examination (i.e. assessing ventricular function, ventricular and atrial size, basic valve function, pericardial and pleural effusions) make transthoracic echocardiography frequently as useful as transoesophageal echocardiography. Such measurements can guide fluid and inotrope therapy (Figures 3 to 6). However, it is important to recognise situations where information may be inconclusive. As with the rest of medicine, there are many situations where experience is important. The echocardiogram alone rarely tells the operator what to do as it only displays what can be seen. The clinical data must be reviewed in the light of the echo findings.

Figure 3. Two chamber transoesophageal view showing a dilated left ventricle.

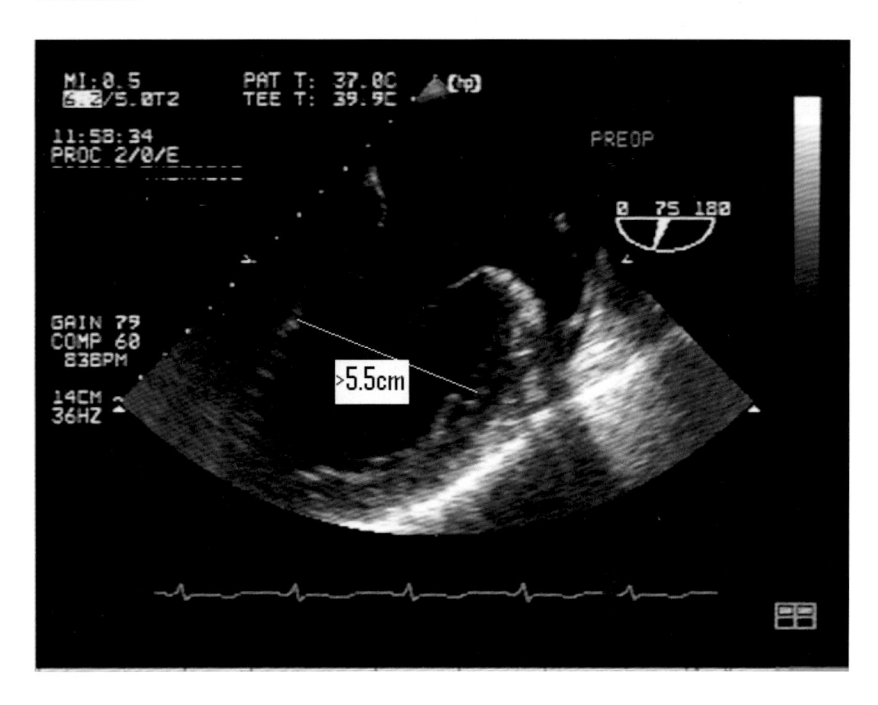

Figure 4. Doppler pattern across the aortic valve showing aortic stenosis.

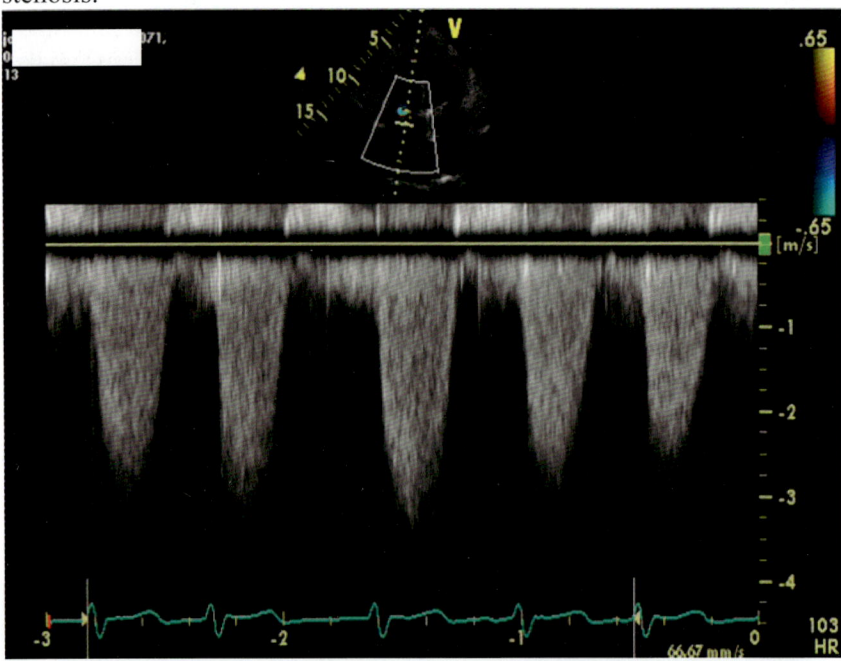

Figure 5. Short axis view of the aortic valve is used for planimetry

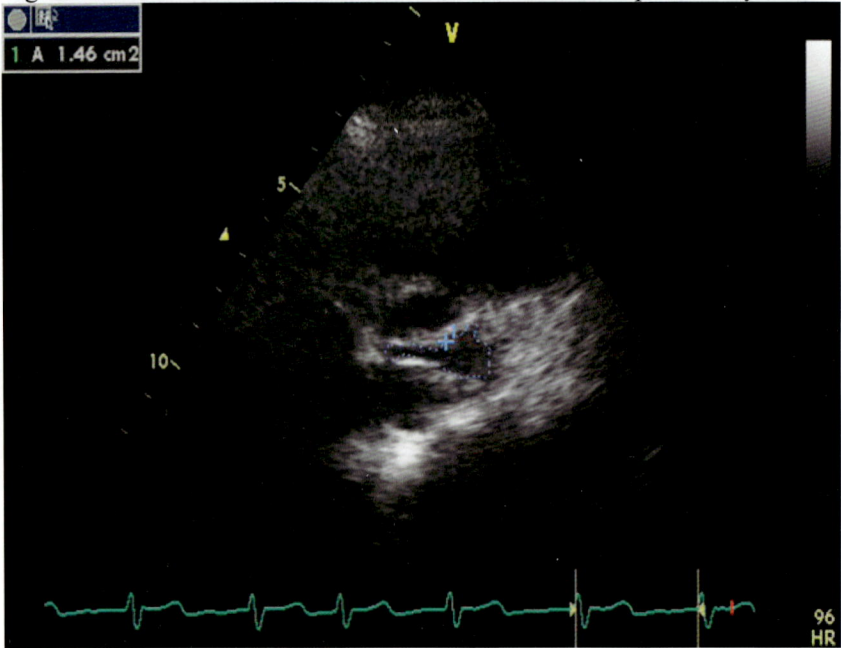

ECHOCARDIOGRAPHY IN THE INTENSIVE CARE UNIT

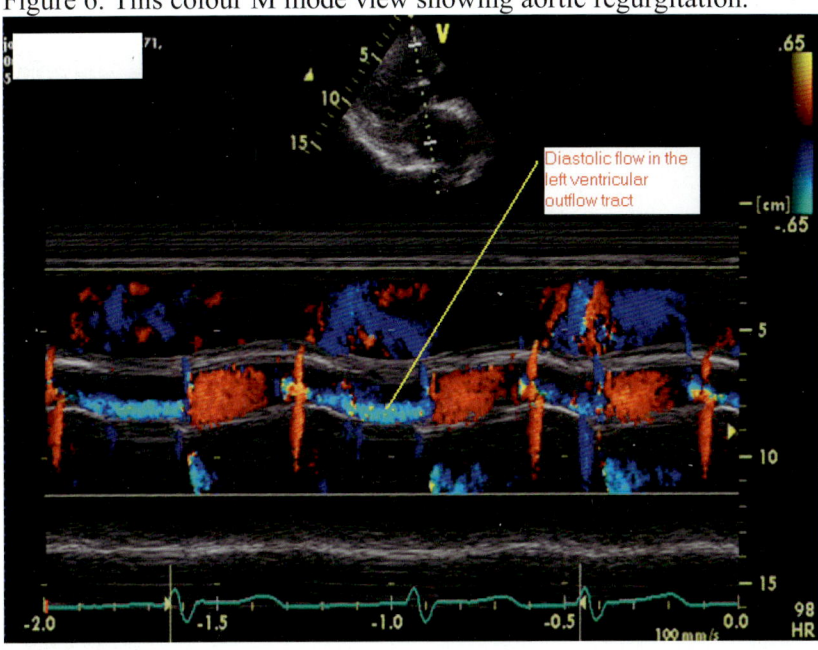

Figure 6. This colour M mode view showing aortic regurgitation.

Figure 7. This rather poor transthoracic echocardiograph shows a small anterior pericardial effusion.

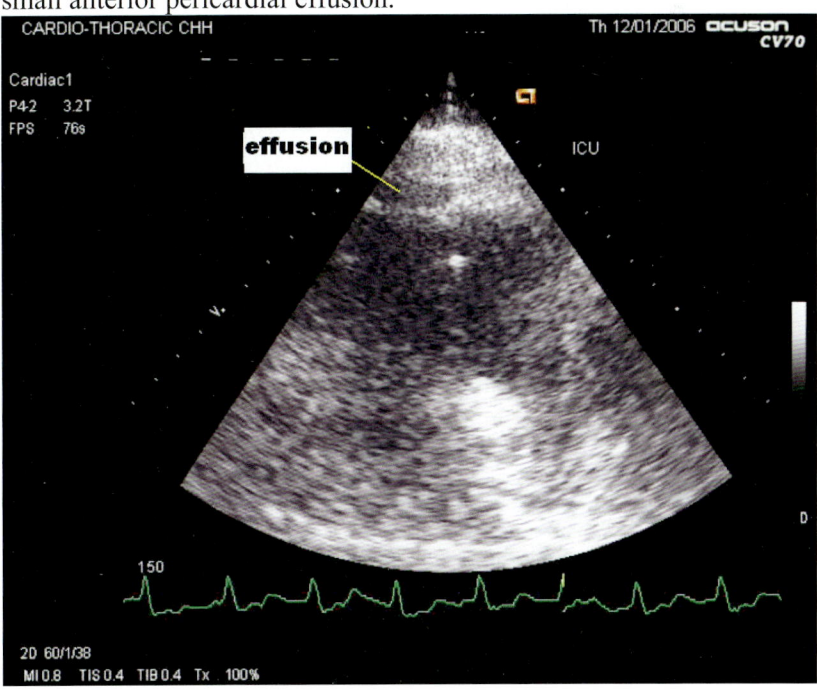

CRITICAL CARE FOCUS 14: UPDATES

Figure 8. This two chamber transthoracic view shows that the pericardial effusion can also been seen along the lateral cardiac border.

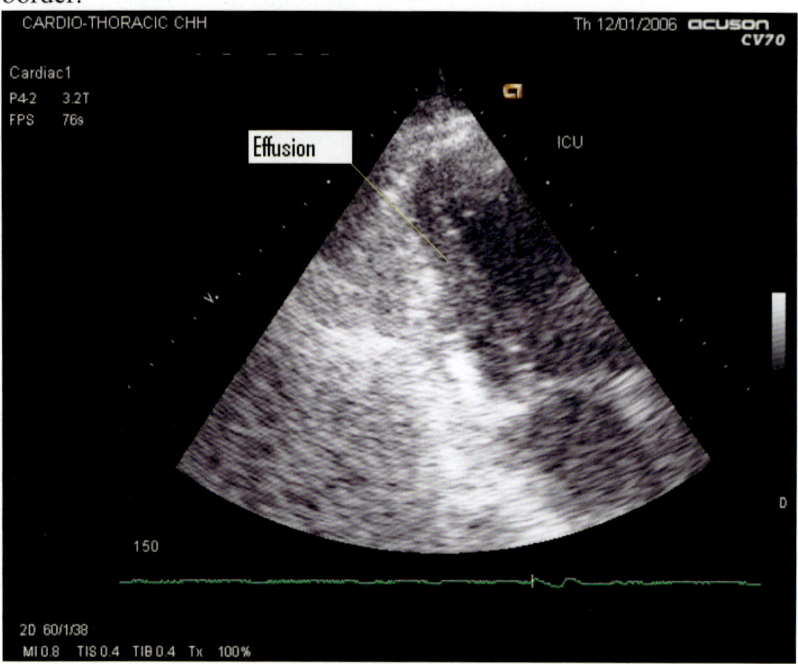

For example, Figures 7 and 8 show rather poor quality transthoracic echocardiography images of a 1 cm pericardial effusion anteriorly and even smaller effusion laterally. The patient was extubated 6 hours after coronary surgery and had a sternal dressing and drains. His haemoglobin level fell and his systolic arterial pressure was below 100 mmHg with a central venous pressure less than 10 cmH$_2$O. Figure 9 showed a large pleural effusion. During drainage of the pleural effusion, the patient collapsed and required re-intubation and immediate chest opening. There was a significant volume of blood in the pericardium but tamponade was not evident as blood was leaking into the pleura. Earlier exploration may have avoided the haemodynamic collapse but the transthoracic echocardiography had just showed where the blood was escaping and not the true underlying problem.

Another patient 3 weeks after colostomy closure was found to have *Methicillin Resistant Staphylococcus aureas* A on the tip of the central catheter. A transthoracic echocardiography suggested that the patient had thrombus or endocarditis visible in the left atrium. A transoesophageal echocardiograph showed a vegetation on the mitral valve (Figure 10).

Figure 9. This transthoracic view shows a significant right pleural effusion.

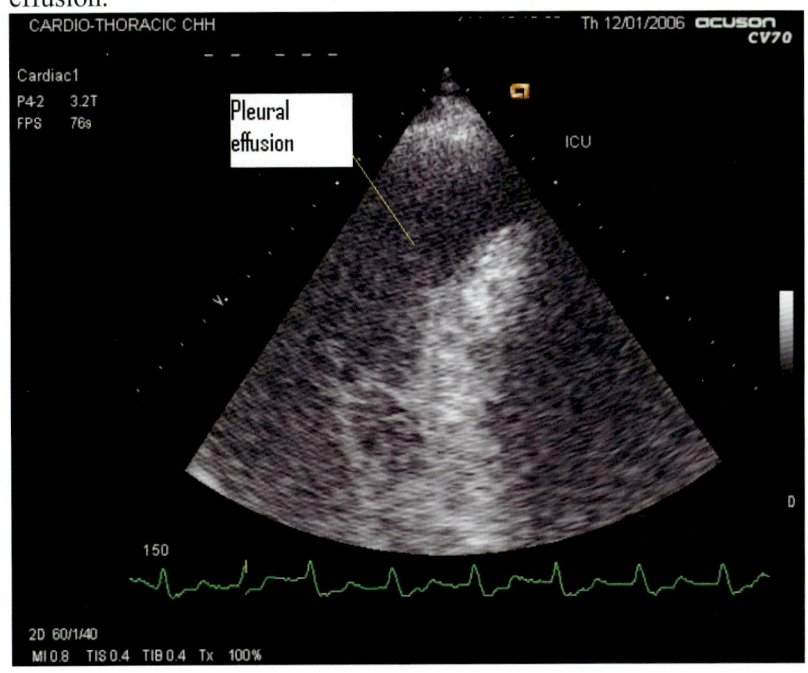

Figure 10. Transoesophageal echocardiograph of the left ventricle using 2 D with Doppler colour showing a vegetation.

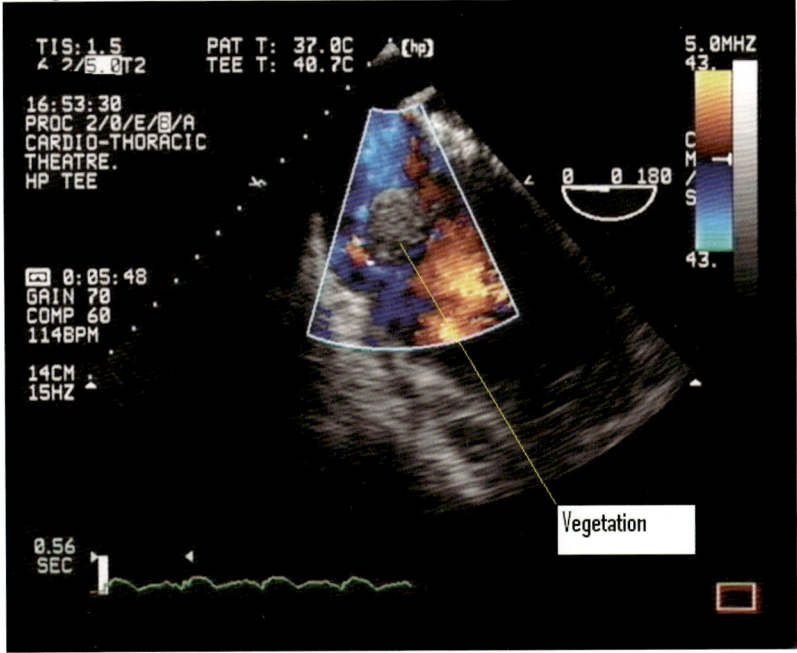

CRITICAL CARE FOCUS 14: UPDATES

Transthoracic echocardiography will frequently be adequate but for exclusion of thrombi, vegetations, ventricular or atrial septal defects or aortic dissection transoesophageal echocardiography is required.

Transoesophageal echocardiography in the critically ill

It is important to have a thorough knowledge of ultrasound based on the standard views [6] and how each view may be used with the different modalities such as colour Doppler, M-mode, etc. Even transoesophageal echocardiography does not always provide good acoustic windows and unexpected findings are common.

The American College of Cardiology with the American Heart Association and the American Society of Echocardiography jointly published practice guidelines for echocardiography [7]. Section XIII deals with 'Echocardiography in the Critically Ill.' This section includes the trauma patient on intensive care. Class 1 indications for the use of echocardiography are haemodynamically unstable patients and patients with suspected aortic dissection. Also included are patients with previous or suspected valve disease. Using these guidelines and various other references, it is possible for the intensivist to have a number of indications for echocardiography as a first line diagnostic and monitoring tool:

1. Hypotension and haemodynamic optimisation
On the surgical wards there may be a general assumption that patients less than seventy years old have good left ventricular function. Thus treatment of hypotension in younger patients focuses on fluid therapy. On the medical ward there is a tendency to give too little fluid for fear of causing pulmonary oedema and subsequent renal dysfunction may have developed. Echocardiography may help the differential diagnosis and guide therapy. On ICU, transoesophageal echocardiography can rationalise inotrope usage and could be considered essential in up to 34% of patients [8].

2. Evaluation of aortic dissection

3. Suspected endocarditis

4. Assessment of valve function

5. Complications of acute myocardial infarction
Left ventricular contractility can be assessed by wall movement, ventricular diameter and fractional area change. Regional wall motion abnormalities suggest ischaemia and end diastolic area is a reliable marker of preload.

6. *Assessment of pericardial / pleural fluid*

7. *Hypoxaemia*
The pulmonary artery can be visualised above the bifurcation. Also thrombi in other chambers can be detected [9].

8. *Source of systemic embolism*

9. *Chest trauma*
Judgement is required to assess the significance of pericardial effusions but when transoesophageal echocardiography data is combined with clinical information nearly 100% success is achieved [10]. Pleural effusions are usually detectable by transthoracic echocardiography but are often a finding during transoesophageal echocardiography in sick patients. Intervention gives good results with low morbidity compared to X-ray [11].

Haemodynamic monitoring
Transoesophageal echocardiography allows more detailed measurements to be made.

Cardiac Output (CO) can be measured using this formula:

CO (ml/min) = time velocity integral (cm) x cross-sectional area (cm^2) x heart rate.

Where the time velocity integral is measured as the aortic flow envelope using pulse wave Doppler in the aortic transgastric view or one of the over outflow areas. Cross-sectional area is measured as the radius at that point.

Ejection fraction (EF)
The area of the left ventricle can be measured in systole and diastole using the long axis view; then by applying Simpson's rule, a volume can be calculated giving ejection fraction (EF).

$$EF (\%) = \frac{\text{End Diastolic volume} - \text{End Systolic volume}}{\text{End Diastolic volume}}$$

Fractional area change (FAC)
This is measured in the transgastric view of the left ventricle. The percent change in systolic and diastolic area equates closely to the ejection fraction.

$$FAC = \frac{\text{End Diastolic area} - \text{End Systolic area}}{\text{End Diastolic area}}$$

Fractional shortening (FS)
This is the excursion of the endocardium in systole and diastole and relates to ejection fraction but is more prone to errors due to regional variations of the myocardium. It is frequently quoted during transthoracic echocardiography examination and many echo machines will use this to calculate ejection fraction. It equates to half the ejection fraction.

$$FS = \frac{\text{End Diastolic diameter} - \text{End Systolic diameter}}{\text{End Diastolic diameter}}$$

These measurements are useful in more complex cases where they may follow the progress of an individual or where objective data is required. While these measurements have been shown to be reliable [12], not all correlate well with conventional monitoring such as the pulmonary artery catheter [13].

Typically the indications for use are more common on a cardiac rather than a general unit. The equipment is expensive as is the cost of training staff and so while justifiable on a cardiac unit, echocardiography may not be so on a general unit.

On a general ICU, admission of a trauma patient is often an indication for transoesophageal echocardiography, with reports suggesting that all penetrating and severe chest trauma should have a transoesophageal echocardiograph [14]. The types of pathology detected are pericardial effusion, pleural effusion, valvular damage, ascending and descending aortic rupture. These findings may not be detected by other diagnostic modalities.

One report in a 24 bedded general ICU performing 308 studies over four years found hypotension (40%) the commonest indication followed by suspected endocarditis (27%), left ventricular function (15%), pulmonary oedema (5%) and suspected thrombus (4%). Aortic and valve pathologies account for less than 10% of cases [15]. Another study categorised non-cardiac ICU patients according to level 1, 2 or 3 indications and found that for level 1 indications (haemodynamic instability and suspected aortic pathology) transoesophageal echocardiography altered management in 60% of cases [16].

ECHOCARDIOGRAPHY IN THE INTENSIVE CARE UNIT

Some centres have reported that transthoracic echocardiography is not cost effective because of the capital outlay and training costs for staff who are not spending the majority of their time performing echocardiography [17]. Also transoesophageal echocardiography is more reliable on ICU in over 65% of patients studied [18]. However as technology improves this may change and as Jensen points out one often only needs one good view with transthoracic echocardiography to provide the desired information.

Training in Echocardiography
On most general critical care units ultrasound in general, and echocardiography in particular, is underused. This is at least in part due to the services that perform the studies not having dedicated ICU time and when the staff arrive they are not experts in intensive care. A recent editorial by Bodenham [19] pointed out the lack of accredited training available in the UK with the exception of echocardiography. The Association of Cardiothoracic Anaesthetists (ACTA) (www.acta.org.uk) currently provide practical training in transoesophageal echocardiography. The British Society of Echocardiography (BSE) (www.bsecho.org) run similar transthoracic echocardiography courses. Accreditation in transoesophageal echocardiography is via the British Society of Echocardiography / Association of Cardiothoracic Anaesthetists joint accreditation which involves an examination and a logbook. Accreditation in transthoracic echocardiography is similar and run by the British Society of Echocardiography. Both also require evidence of continuing practice for re-accreditation and set a standard which would allow intensivists to feel competent using echocardiography on ICU.

For the intensivist, competence in transoesophageal and transthoracic echocardiography would be appropriate because the information is needed 24 hours a day and would combine diagnosis with monitoring. This would be goal directed ultrasound examining vascular anatomy (including heart valves), effusions, left ventricular function and circulating volume management. While both transoesophageal and transthoracic echocardiography are similar in many respects, obtaining accreditation in both would be a lengthy process. To date, most anaesthetists have opted for transoesophageal echocardiography due to access to cardiac patients. However, transthoracic echocardiography can be very useful on ICU.

For the awake patient, level 2 transthoracic echocardiography is required. The sonographer should have the British Society of Echocardiography transthoracic echocardiography accreditation.

A different level of training for intensive care is not currently available and would require collaboration between the existing societies. A training package including a wide range of ultrasound applications may be attractive to intensivists.

Conclusion
In the few cases where conventional monitoring has failed, transthoracic and transoesophageal echocardiography can provide rapid, safe information that has been shown to alter management. Now we need to learn how to use echocardiography properly and assess outcomes.

References
1. McLean AS. Transoesophageal echocardigraphy in the intensive care unit. Anaesthesia and Intensive Care 1998; 26: 22-25.
2. Townend JN, Hutton P. Transeosophageal echocardiography and intensive care. British Journal of Anaesthesia 1996; 77: 137-9.
3. Poelaert J, Schmidt C. Transoesophageal echocardiography in the critically ill. Anaesthesia 1998; 53: 55-68.
4. Goswami S, Weller M. Usefulness of hand-carried echographic devices in perioperative medicine. Anesthesia and Analgesia 2004; 98: SCA25.
5. Jensen MB, Sloth E. Echocardiography in intensive care. Acta Anaesthesia Scandinavia 2004; 48: 1069-1070.
6. Shanewise JS, Cheung AT, Aronson S. ASE/SCA Guidelines for performing a Comprehensive Intraop TOE: Task Force recommendations. Anesthesia and Analgesia 1999; 89: 870-884.
7. Cheitlin MD, Armstrong WF, Aurigemma GP, *et al.* ACC/AHA/ASE 2003 Guideline Update for the Clinical Application of Echocardiography: summary article. Journal of the American Society of Echocardiography 2003; 16: 1091-1110.
8. Costachescu T, Denault A. The hemodynamically unstable patient in the ICU: hemodynamic vs TOE monitoring. Critical Care Medicine 2002; 30: 1214-1223.
9. Vieillard BA, Qanadli SD. TOE for the diagnosis of pulmonary embolism with acute *cor pulmonale*: a comparison with radiological procedures. Intensive Care Medicine 1998; 24: 429-33.
10. Bommer WJ, Follette D. Tamponade in patients undergoing cardiac surgery: a clinical-echocardographic diagnosis. American Heart Journal 1995; 130: 1216-23.
11. Diacon AH, Martin H. Accuracy of pleural puncture sites. Chest 2003; 123: 436-441.

12. Fontes ML, Bellows W. Assessment of ventricular function in critically ill patients: limitations of PA catheter. Journal of Cardiothoracic and Vascular Anesthesia 1999; 13: 521-527.
13. Bouchard MJ, Denault A. Poor correlation between hemodynamic and echocardiographic indexes of left ventricular performance in the operating room and ICU. Critical Care Medicine 2004; 32: 644-648.
14. Porembka DT, Johnson DJ. Penetrating cardiac trauma: a perioperative role for TOE. Anesthesia and Analgesia 1993; 77: 1275-1277.
15. Colreavy FB, Donovan K. TOE in critically ill patients. Critical Care Medicine 2002; 30: 989-996.
16. Denault AY, Couture P. Perioperative use of TOE by anesthesiologists: impact in non-cardiac surgery and ICU. Canadian Journal of Anaesthesia 2002; 49: 287-293.
17. Cook CH, Praba AC. Transthoracic echocardiography is not cost-effective in critically ill surgical patients. Journal of Trauma 202; 52: 280-284.
18. Slama MA, Novara A. Diagnostic and therapeutic implications of TOE in medical ICU patients with unexplained shock, hypoxemia or suspected endocarditis. Intensive Care Medicine 1996; 22: 916-22.
19. Bodenham AR. Ultrasound imaging by anaesthetists: training and accreditation issues. British Journal of Anaesthesia 2006; 96: 414-417.

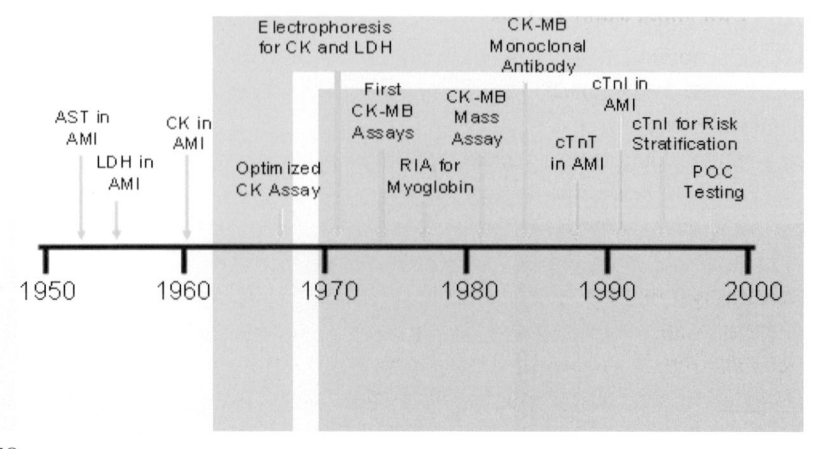

5: Biomarkers in Acute Coronary Syndrome – Introducing Heart-Fatty Acid-Binding Protein (H-FABP)

DR NIAMH KILCULLEN and PROF ALISTAIR HALL

History of markers in the diagnosis of myocardial infarction
The diagnosis of myocardial infarction hinges on the combination of biochemical markers, clinical features and ECG changes. Cardiac markers have played an important role in the diagnosis and management of acute myocardial infarction since 1954 when aspartate aminotransferase assays were introduced (Figure 1). Asparate aminotransferase is normally found in liver, heart, muscle, kidney and brain. It is released into serum when any one of these tissues is damaged. In 1965, creatinine kinase was identified as a useful marker for diagnosing myocardial infarction as it is more muscle specific. However, creatinine kinase is found in skeletal, smooth and cardiac muscle and is released into the bloodstream following any muscle damage. Serum creatinine kinase increases within 4-8 hrs of an acute myocardial infarction and so is able to assist in the early diagnosis of myocardial infarction.

Figure 1. History of cardiac markers (AST: asparate aminotransferase, LDH: lactate dehydrogenase, CK: creatinine kinase, AMI: acute myocardial infarction, CK-MB: creatinine kinase-myocardium bound, RIA: radioimmunoassay, cTn: cardiac troponin, POC: point of care)

Troponin

Cardiac troponin is a complex molecule composed of three different polypeptides all of which are involved in myocyte contraction. The first of these, troponin I, prevents muscle contraction in the absence of calcium; troponin T connects the troponin complex to tropomyosin and troponin C binds calcium. Numerous studies have demonstrated that elevated cardiac troponins in patients with suspected acute coronary syndromes predict adverse outcomes (i.e. death and non-fatal myocardial infarction) during both short- and long-term follow-up studies [1–3]. A meta-analysis of 21 studies of patients with suspected acute coronary syndromes demonstrated an odds ratio for death and myocardial infarction at 30 days of 3.44 (95% confidence interval (CI) 2.94 – 4.03; $p<0.001$) for troponin-positive patients [4]. Troponin immunoassays (both I and T) are now widely accepted as providing a valuable guide to diagnosis and risk stratification for patients with acute coronary syndromes [5].

Limitations of cardiac troponins

Cardiac troponins have some limitations in patients with suspected acute coronary syndrome. Many non-ischaemic pathologies can cause myocardial necrosis (Table 1) and therefore elevations in cardiac troponin concentrations [6].

Table 1. Non-ischaemic cardiac pathologies raising serum cardiac troponin.

Acute rheumatic fever
Amyloidosis
Cardiac trauma
Cardiotoxicity
Congestive heart failure
Critical illness (including sepsis)
End stage renal failure
Glycogen storage disease type II
Heart transplantation
Haemoglobinopathy
Hypertension or Hypotension
Myocarditis and / or pericarditis
Pulmonary embolism

Secondly, among the 15 or so available assays for troponin I, imprecision at low concentrations can give false-positive results [7]. The consensus definition for myocardial infarction defined a threshold value for cardiac troponin as a measurement exceeding the 99th percentile of a reference control group. Acceptable imprecision at the

99th percentile for each assay was defined as ≤ 10%. However, Panteghini *et al* [8] found that no commercial assay could achieve a 10% coefficient of variation at the 99th percentile reference limit so failing to differentiate between minor myocardial injury and analytical error.

Finally, troponins achieve their greatest sensitivity and specificity 10-12 hrs after symptom onset and may therefore be falsely negative when measured earlier in admission. While the 12-lead ECG is a useful tool in early risk stratification, difficulties arise when the ECGs are non-diagnostic (e.g. left bundle branch block, paced rhythm) or persistently abnormal from previous myocardial infarctions. Even among patients with a normal 12-lead ECG, a subsequent diagnosis of myocardial infarction can still be confirmed in 6% of patients [9].

Literature data on the prognosis of patients with suspected acute coronary syndrome and negative troponins is limited and inconsistent. The largest published follow-up study is from Finland with 764 patients discharged from hospital after 24 hrs of observation, two negative troponins (6-12 hrs apart) and no progressive ECG changes. This study reported a 6-month all-cause mortality of 2.3% [10]. However other studies report a high rate of major adverse cardiac events (e.g. myocardial infarction, the need for revascularization, or death) among troponin-negative patients [11]. Dudek *et al* [12] studied 104 patients admitted with class IIIB unstable angina pectoris (i.e. angina occurring at rest and presenting within 48 hrs) and noted no difference in major adverse cardiac events between troponin positive and negative groups after follow-up for 30 days.

Therefore an additional early marker to facilitate appropriate triage of patients with suspected acute coronary syndrome and identify those suitable for aggressive interventions is needed. A variety of novel biomarkers are currently under evaluation of which heart-fatty acid-binding protein is one.

Fatty acid-binding proteins
Cytoplasmic fatty acid-binding proteins (FABP) are a group of at least 13 low molecular weight proteins involved in lipid homeostasis. They facilitate the cytoplasmic translocation of long chain fatty acids [13] and are found in a number of tissues including liver (L-FABP), intestine (I-FABP), heart (H-FABP) and brain (B-FABP). Fatty acid-binding proteins were previously regarded as merely intracellular equivalents of plasma albumin but recent reports suggest they may have other important roles in signal transduction, cell growth and differentiation and possibly cytoprotection [14]. These proteins

contain between 126-137 amino acid residues and show an amino acid sequence homology of 20-70%. Each protein consists of two α-helices and 10 anti-parallel (i.e. amino sequences running in opposite directions) β-strands, organised in two β-sheets forming a clam shell-like structure. Binding of the fatty acids occurs inside the molecule by interaction with various amino acids within the binding pocket or β-barrel of the protein [15] (Figure 2).

Heart-fatty acid-binding protein
Heart-fatty acid-binding protein is primarily expressed in cardiac myocytes (0.5 mg/g wet weight) [16] but is also found in skeletal muscle (0.05 – 0.2mg/g wet weight [17], distal tubule of the kidneys [18] and brain tissue [19]. The heart-fatty acid-binding protein gene is located on chromosome 1 (1p32-1p33) [20]. In 1985 Glatz [21] isolated heart fatty acid-binding protein from human hearts and reported its molecular weight as 15 kDa and isoelectric point (pI) as 7.5. He later found that heart-fatty acid-binding protein contains 132 amino acids and is an acidic protein (pI 5) [22]. However, it has been suggested that different isoforms of heart-fatty acid-binding protein exist within the human heart. In 1986, Unterberg et al [23] isolated heart-fatty acid-binding protein from human cardiac tissue with a molecular weight of 15.5 kDa and an isoelectric point of 5.3.

Immunochemical assays of heart-fatty acid-binding protein
A large number of immunoassays using both monoclonal and polyclonal antibodies have been developed. Most of the assays available are enzyme-linked immunosorbent assays (ELISA) [24, 25]. Monoclonal antibodies are now generally used as these show almost no cross-reactivity with other fatty acid-binding protein types [26]. Recombinant heart-fatty acid-binding protein can be used as a standard in immunoassays as it appears to behave immunochemically in the same way as tissue derived heart-fatty acid-binding protein [24]. The drawback of these assays is the time it takes to analyse samples as the quickest immunoassay available currently takes 45 mins. In 2001, a simple whole blood panel test for detection of heart-fatty acid-binding protein within 15 mins was developed using one-step immunochromatography [27]. This test is designed for point of care testing and identifies patients with heart-fatty acid-binding protein concentrations greater than 6 μg/l. More recently there has been interest in developing biosensors for detection of heart-fatty acid-binding protein in plasma. The ideal fatty acid-binding protein biosensor for bedside monitoring would allow continuous monitoring of heart-fatty acid-binding protein thereby assisting the clinician in distinguishing minor myocardial infarctions from unstable angina [28].

Figure 2. Structure of heart fatty acid binding protein (modified from: Lucke C, Huang S, Rademacher M, Ruterjans H. New insights into intracellular lipid binding proteins: The role of buried water. Protein Science 2002; 11: 2382-2392 with permission)

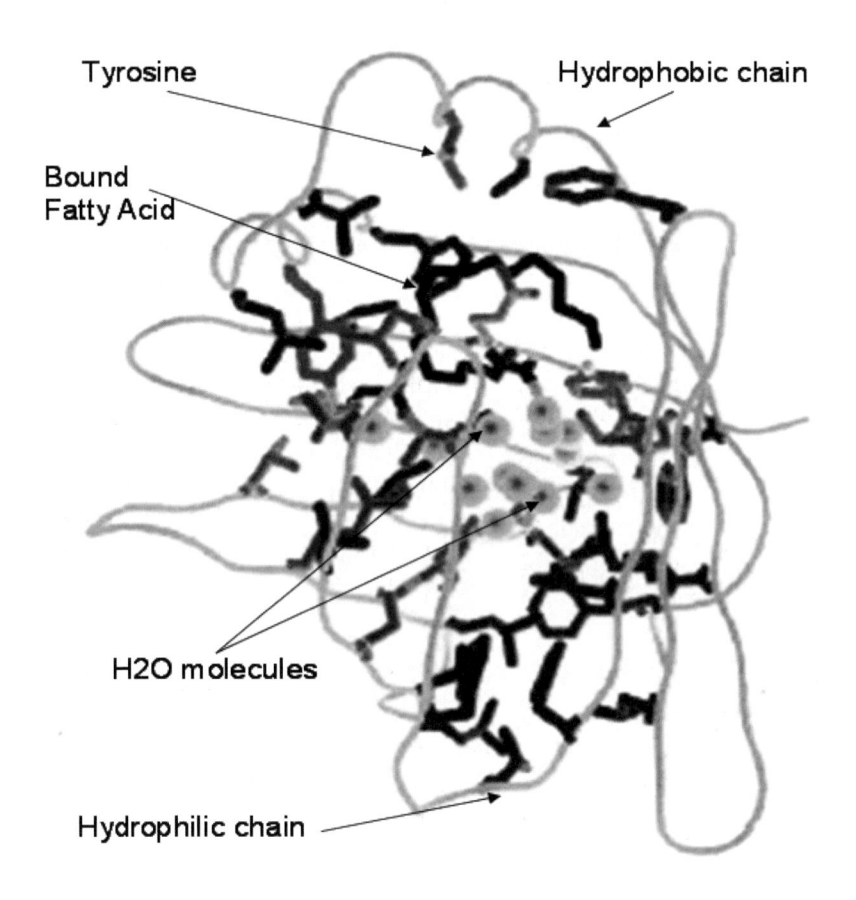

Reference limits for assays are often derived from concentrations found in healthy controls. Typically the 97.5th (mean ± 2 standard deviations (SD)) or 99th (mean ± 3 SD) percentiles are used in determining the reference range. Upper reference limits are variable but 6 µg/l has been proposed by Pelsers *et al* [29] and Pagani *et al* [30]. Heart-fatty acid-binding protein is renally excreted and can be detected in urine within 3 hrs following acute myocardial infarction [31]. Górski *et al* [32] found markedly elevated heart-fatty acid-binding protein concentrations in 27 patients with chronic renal failure and therefore in the setting of an acute myocardial infarction, it is likely that the pre-infarct concentration may already be elevated if the patient has chronic renal impairment.

Biological variability of heart fatty acid-binding protein

Pelsers *et al* [29] reported the effect of age, sex and day-to-day fluctuations on heart-fatty acid-binding protein concentrations in healthy controls. Heart-fatty acid-binding protein concentrations varied slightly depending on the time of day but overall such variation was not thought to be significant. More importantly, plasma heart-fatty acid-binding protein increases with age, presumably reflecting the age-related decrease in renal function. Men have higher concentrations of heart-fatty acid-binding protein because of their relatively larger muscle mass.

Heart-fatty acid-binding protein and myocardial disease

Heart-fatty acid-binding protein is rapidly released from the cytosol following cell ischaemia and necrosis and was first isolated from injured myocardium in 1988 [33]. Since then, heart-fatty acid-binding protein has been shown to be a sensitive and potentially useful early marker of myocardial infarction [34-36]. The release kinetics of heart-fatty acid-binding protein post myocardial infarction are well established; it is typically detectable at 1-3 hrs, peaks at 6-8 hrs and returns to baseline concentrations at 24-30 hrs [37]. Interestingly, thrombolysis therapy does not affect the release ratio of heart fatty acid-binding protein but an accelerated protein release rate is observed [38].

Rationale for heart-fatty acid-binding protein as early marker of myocardial injury

Heart-fatty acid-binding protein has many advantages over other cardiac markers since it is confined to the cytoplasm and has a small molecular size that facilitates early release following myocardial ischaemia. It is similar to myoglobin which is an established early marker of myocardial infarction; however, it is important to acknowledge that elevated concentrations are not synonymous with myocardial damage as heart-fatty acid-binding protein is also found in skeletal muscle. The heart-fatty acid-binding protein content in skeletal muscle is only 10-30% of that found in the myocardium [39]. On the other hand, the skeletal muscle content of myoglobin is twice that of cardiac muscle [16]. Heart-fatty acid-binding protein has been shown to increase 13.9 fold after physical exercise in otherwise healthy subjects [40] and elevated concentrations may also be observed following cardioversion, post-operatively or in multi-organ failure [41]. The presence of heart-fatty acid-binding protein in skeletal muscle is a potential drawback for diagnosing myocardial injury. However, in order to differentiate between myocardial and skeletal injury, the plasma myoglobin / heart-fatty acid-binding protein ratio has been proposed [16]. The ratio in heart muscle is reported as 2 to 10 and 20 to 70 in skeletal muscle; therefore, a lower myoglobin / heart fatty acid-binding protein ratio favours a cardiac source.

Heart-fatty acid-binding protein and unstable angina
A few studies have examined the role of heart-fatty acid-binding protein in patients presenting with unstable angina who often have minor degrees of myocardial injury. Katrukha *et al* [42] measured serial concentrations of heart-fatty acid-binding protein (with the HyTest (HyTest, Intelligate 6th floor, Joukahaisenkatu 6, 20520, Turku, Finland)) and troponin 1 in 31 patients admitted with unstable angina. Samples were obtained on admission and then at 6, 12, 18 and 24 hrs after the onset of chest pain. A cut-off value of 6 µg/l was used for heart-fatty acid-binding protein. On admission, 54% of patients had elevated concentrations of heart-fatty acid-binding protein compared with 13% with elevated troponin 1 concentrations. Six hours after the onset of chest pain, the proportion with positive tests rose to 58% for heart-fatty acid-binding protein and 52% for troponin 1 indicating that sequential measurements of both markers could be useful in the early diagnosis of minor myocardial injury. Another study examined serum concentrations of heart-fatty acid-binding protein in 15 patients with unstable angina, 19 patients with stable angina and 20 controls. Elevated concentrations of heart-fatty acid-binding protein were observed in the patient group with unstable angina suggesting a useful role for assessing patients with unstable angina [43]. A more recent study measured serum and pericardial concentrations of heart-fatty acid-binding protein in patients with and without unstable angina pre-operatively. Pericardial fluid concentrations were significantly higher in patients with unstable angina reflecting myocardial ischaemia [44].

Heart-fatty acid-binding protein and myocardial infarction
Several studies have shown that heart-fatty acid-binding protein is an excellent early marker of myocardial infarction [21,34,36,39]. The majority of studies such as the multi-centre EUROCARDI study have compared the diagnostic performance of heart-fatty acid-binding protein with myoglobin. A subgroup of patients admitted within three hours after the onset of symptoms showed an area under the receiver operating characteristic curve of 0.845 for heart-fatty acid-binding protein and 0.717 for myoglobin. A subgroup of patients admitted 3-6 hrs after the onset of symptoms had an area under the receiver operating characteristic curve of 0.945 for heart-fatty acid-binding protein and 0.892 for myoglobin [35]. Okamoto *et al* [34] compared the diagnostic accuracy of heart-fatty acid-binding protein with

creatinine kinase-myocardium bound and myoglobin and concluded that:

> "....heart-fatty acid-binding protein has excellent diagnostic accuracy for the detection of myocardial damage within 12 hours, and even within 3 hours".

Patients with suspected acute myocardial infarction within 12 hrs after the onset of symptoms showed an area under the receiver operating characteristic curve of 0.921 for heart-fatty acid-binding protein, 0.843 for myoglobin and 0.654 for creatinine kinase-myocardium bound. At least 12 studies comparing the diagnostic performance of heart-fatty acid-binding protein and myoglobin have been reported and in general conclude that heart-fatty acid-binding protein is a superior early marker of myocardial infarction. A study by Ghani *et al* [45] examined heart-fatty acid-binding protein, myoglobin, creatinine kinase-myocardium bound and troponin I in 460 patients presenting with chest pain and reported a low sensitivity and specificity for heart-fatty acid-binding protein. However on closer inspection, this discrepancy is explained by the fact that samples were timed from admission and not onset of symptoms as in other studies.

A second study by Alansari and Croal [46] in 2004 assessed the clinical value of heart-fatty acid-binding protein and myoglobin in addition to troponin I in patients presenting with chest pain. Blood samples were taken on admission and again at 12 hrs. Greater receiver operating characteristic curve areas were obtained for troponin I over both heart-fatty acid-binding protein and myoglobin. It is worth pointing out that the median time from onset of symptoms was 5 hrs (interquartile range (IQR) 3 – 12 hrs) and the authors acknowledge that this may have influenced the results. It is well recognised that determining the exact time of onset of symptoms can be difficult and therefore many studies time blood samples from admission rather than the onset of chest pain. As heart-fatty acid-binding protein is an early marker of myocardial infarction, it is extremely important that the onset of symptoms is clearly identified so that samples are taken at the appropriate time. It has been suggested that serial samples of heart-fatty acid-binding protein may improve the diagnostic accuracy in patients suspected of myocardial infarction [47].

Heart-fatty acid-binding protein and infarct size / reperfusion / reinfarction
The measurement of infarct size is not routinely performed although it does have important prognostic implications [48,49]. Glatz *et al* compared the release of heart-fatty acid-binding protein, creatinine

kinase-myocardium bound and hydroxybutyrate dehydrogenase into plasma after myocardial infarction and estimated infarct size from corresponding plasma curves. They reported that a clinically useful estimate of myocardial size could be given provided frequent blood samples were taken for heart-fatty acid-binding protein concentrations [49]. Wodzig et al [50] recommended that heart-fatty acid-binding protein could be used to estimate infarct size but only if renal function was normal as heart infarct size may be overestimated in patients with renal dysfunction. This problem was addressed by de Groot et al [51] who reported that by using individually estimated renal clearance rates, heart-fatty acid-binding protein can be used to estimate myocardial damage and infarct size within 24 hrs of symptoms.

Some studies have shown that heart fatty acid-binding protein is a sensitive and specific marker of coronary reperfusion [52,53]. Both heart-fatty acid-binding protein and myoglobin concentrations rise sharply following successful reperfusion whereas they rise more slowly if reperfusion has failed. Abe et al [54] reported that a rise in the heart-fatty acid-binding protein ratio of 1.5 or more (compared to pre-treatment concentration) as an index of reperfusion demonstrated an accuracy of 100% after 30 mins and 94% after 60 mins. Re-infarction after myocardial infarction typically presents as further chest pain with or without ECG changes. Cardiac biomarkers are usually not helpful as they are generally already elevated from the initial infarct. However, heart-fatty acid-binding protein with its rapid release kinetics and renal clearance has been shown to accurately diagnose infarction [16].

Heart-fatty acid-binding protein & cardiac failure
It is well recognised that cardiac biomarkers such as troponin T can be elevated in patients with severe heart failure, possibly representing ongoing myocardial damage [55-57]. Elevated concentrations of heart-fatty acid-binding protein have also been reported in patients with chronic heart failure and are associated with subsequent cardiac events [58]. These findings were confirmed in a larger study by Arimoto et al [59] who measured heart-fatty acid-binding protein in 179 patients with congestive heart failure and followed them for 20 months. The cardiac event rate was markedly higher in patients with elevated concentrations of heart-fatty acid-binding protein than in those with normal concentrations (43% versus 7%; $p<0.001$).

Heart-fatty acid-binding protein as a prognostic marker
At present, little is known about the prognostic value of heart-fatty acid-binding protein in patients presenting with acute coronary syndrome. Only a small number of studies have examined the

potential role of heart-fatty acid-binding protein in risk stratification in acute coronary syndrome. A recent study by Nakata et al [60] found heart-fatty acid-binding protein to be equal to myoglobin and superior to troponin T in predicting the early (within 7 days) adverse outcomes such as emergency hospitalisation, emergency coronary angiography or other intervention. Heart-fatty acid-binding protein has an area under the receiver operating characteristic curve of 0.936 for patients with acute coronary syndrome. This was significantly better than was observed for myoglobin, creatinine kinase-myocardium bound and troponin T. The authors suggest that this improved performance is due to the large amount of heart-fatty acid-binding protein present within the cytosol, its greater concentration in myocytes and also its small molecular size (15 kDa) that all facilitate early release.

The only substantial study on the prognostic value of heart-fatty acid-binding protein in acute coronary syndrome was published by Ishii et al [61]. Ishii examined serum troponin T and heart-fatty acid-binding protein in 328 consecutive patients admitted with acute coronary syndrome within 6 hrs after symptom onset. Patients were included if they had within 6 hrs of admission an episode of anginal chest pain lasting over 10 mins and at least one of the following ECG changes: ST elevation or depression (at least 0.05 mV), T wave inversion (at least 0.1 mV in two contiguous leads) or presumed new left bundle branch block. Troponin T and creatinine kinase-myocardium bound were also measured on admission but biochemical markers were not part of the inclusion criteria. Exclusion criteria included revascularisation within 6 months and renal impairment (i.e. creatinine >130 µg/l). During the 6 month follow-up there were 15 cardiac deaths and 10 non-fatal myocardial infarctions. Multivariate analysis examined clinical, electrocardiographic and biochemical variables and revealed that elevated heart-fatty acid-binding protein (median 9.8 µg/l) was independently associated with cardiac events in all patients (relative risk = 9; $p < 0.001$). They concluded that heart-fatty acid-binding protein was independently associated with cardiac death and also cardiac events during 6 months of follow-up. Furthermore heart-fatty acid-binding protein may provide prognostic information in addition to that derived from single measurements of troponin T.

This study used the median value of 9.8 µg/l as a threshold. Cut-off values may also be determined using receiver operating characteristic curve analysis; however, the authors felt it was not appropriate due to the small study size. The decision to use the median value as a cut-off value was justified based on the relatively small number of cardiac events (n = 25). The authors conclude by suggesting that the higher cut-off value has greater prognostic value compared with the established cut-off concentration of 6.2 µg/l for predicting cardiac death and cardiac events. However, they do acknowledge that larger studies are necessary to determine the optimum cut-off value of heart-fatty acid-binding protein.

Two further studies have been published in abstract form. Takeda *et al* [62] measured heart-fatty acid-binding protein in 200 patients presenting to the emergency room with chest symptoms (e.g. chest pain or discomfort, palpitations and dyspnoea) and found that elevated concentrations of heart-fatty acid-binding protein were associated with more cardiac events over the next 7 days. In another small study by Erlikh *et al* [63], heart-fatty acid-binding protein was found to be a prognostic marker of death and non-fatal myocardial infarction in patients with non-ST elevation acute coronary syndrome after 6 months of follow-up.

Conclusion
An ideal marker should be specific to cardiac tissue (i.e. not present in non-cardiac tissue), be released rapidly after injury, and persist in plasma to allow measurement. Assays must have high sensitivity and specificity as well as being rapid and cost effective. Troponin has been shown to have such characteristics and in the late 1980s the first troponin assays were introduced. The availability of cardiac troponin to detect myocardial injury necessitated revision of the diagnostic criteria for myocardial infarction. In 2000, myocardial infarction was redefined by the Joint European Society of Cardiology / American College of Cardiology Committee and the World Health Organisation definition was deemed inappropriate in view of rapid developments in this area. The key areas of progress that resulted in this change were the validation and increasing use of troponin assays in detecting small amounts of myocardial necrosis and the widespread understanding that unstable angina and myocardial infarction represent a single heterogeneous disease state now known as acute coronary syndrome. However, troponin cannot alone describe the full spectrum of pathology, particularly when assessing patients very early after symptom onset and also when cardiac ischaemia dominates over necrosis. In this regard heart-fatty acid-binding protein provides additional valuable information.

References
1) Hamm CW, Ravkilde J, Gerhadt W, *et al*. The prognostic value of serum Troponin T in unstable angina. New England Journal of Medicine 1992; 327: 146-150.
2) Antman E, Tanasijevic M, Thompson B, *et al*. Cardiac-specific troponin I levels to predict the risk of mortality in patients with

acute coronary syndromes. New England Journal of Medicine 1996; 335: 1342-1349.
3) Van Domburg RT, Cobbaert C, Kimman GJ, *et al*. Long-term prognostic value of serial Troponin T bedside tests in patients with acute coronary syndromes. American Journal of Cardiology 2000; 86: 623-627.
4) Ottani F, Galvani M, Nicolini FA, *et al.* Elevated cardiac troponin levels predict the risk of adverse outcome in patients with acute coronary syndromes. American Heart Journal 2000; 140: 917-927.
5) Hamm CW. Acute coronary syndromes. The diagnostic role of troponins. Thrombosis Research 2001; 103: S63-S69.
6) Panteghini M. Role and importance of biochemical markers in clinical cardiology. European Heart Journal 2004; 25: 1187-1196.
7) Apple FS, Quist HE, Doyle PJ, *et al*. Plasma 99th centile reference limits for cardiac troponin and creatinine kinase MB mass for use with European Society of Cardiology/ American College of Cardiology consensus recommendations. Clinical Chemistry 2003; 49: 1331-1336.
8) Panteghini M, Pagani F, Yeo KTJ, *et al* on behalf of the Committee on standardization of markers of cardiac damage of the IFCC. Evaluation of imprecision for cardiac troponin assays at low-range concentrations. Clinical Chemistry 2004; 50: 327-332.
9) Gibler WB, Cannon CP, Blomkalns AL, *et al*. Practical implementation of the guidelines for unstable angina/non-ST-elevation MI in the emergency department. Circulation 2005; 111: 2699-2710.
10) Koukkunen H, Pyörälä K, Halinen MO. Low-risk patients with chest pain and without evidence of myocardial infarction may be safely discharged from emergency department. European Heart Journal 2004; 25: 329-334.
11) Brennan ML, Penn MS, Van Lente F. Prognostic value of myeloperoxidase in patients with chest pain. New England Journal of Medicine 2003; 349: 1595-1604.
12) Dudek D, Chyrchel M, Legutko J, *et al.* Outcomes of patients presenting with acute coronary syndromes and negative Troponin-T. International Journal of Cardiology 2003; 88: 49-55.
13) Schaap FG, Binas B, Danneberg H, van der Vusse GJ, Glatz JFC. Impaired long-chain fatty acid utilization by cardiac myocytes isolated from mice lacking the heart-type fatty acid binding protein gene. Circulation Research 1999; 85: 329-337.
14) Glatz JFC and van der Vusse GJ. Cellular fatty acid-binding proteins: their function and physiological significance. Progress in Lipid Research 1996; 35: 243-282.
15) Banaszak L, Winter N, Xu Z, Bernlohr DA, Cowan S, Jones TA. Lipid-binding proteins: A family of fatty acid and retinoid

transport proteins. Advances in Protein Chemistry 1994; 45: 89-151.
16) Van Nieuwenhoven FA, Kleine AH, Wodzig WH, et al. Discrimination between myocardial and skeletal muscle injury by assessment of the plasma ratio of myoglobin over fatty acid-binding protein. Circulation 1995; 92: 2848-2854.
17) Yoshimoto K, Tanaka T, Somiya K, et al. Human heart-type cytoplasmic fatty-acid binding protein as an indicator of acute myocardial infarction. Heart Vessels 1995; 10: 304-309.
18) Maatman RG, van de Westerlo EM, van Kuppevelt TH, Veerkamp JH. Molecular identification of the liver- and the heart-type fatty acid-binding proteins in human and rat kidney. Use of the reverse transcriptase polymerase chain reaction. Biochemical Journal 1992; 288: 285-290.
19) Pelsers MM, Hanhoff T, van der Voort D, et al. Tissue specific types of fatty acid-binding proteins, B- and H-FABP, as novel markers for detection of brain injury. Clinical Chemistry 2000; 50: 1568-1575.
20) Troxler RF, Offner GD, Jiang J-W, et al. Localization of the gene for human heart fatty acid binding protein to chromosome 1p32-1p33. Human Genetics 1993; 92: 563-566.
21) Glatz JF, Paulussen RJ, Veerkamp JH. Fatty acid binding protein from heart. Chemistry and Physics of Lipids 1985; 38: 115-129.
22) Glatz JFC, van der Voort D, Hermens WT. Fatty acid-binding protein as the earliest available plasma marker of acute myocardial injury. Journal of Clinical Ligand Assay. 2005; 25: 167-177.
23) Unterberg C, Heidl G, Von Bassewitz DB, Spener F. Isolation and characterization of fatty acid-binding protein from human heart. Journal of Lipid Research 1986; 27: 1287-1293.
24) Wodzig KW, Pelsers MM, van der Vusse GJ, Roos W, Glatz JF. One-step enzyme-linked immunosorbent assay (ELISA) for plasma fatty acid-binding protein. Annals of Clinical Biochemistry 1997; 34: 263-268.
25) Ohkaru Y, Tanaka T, Kitaura Y, et al. Point-of-care testing of H-FABP for the diagnosis of acute myocardial infarction: Comparison with conventional tests for myoglobin, CK-MB and troponin T. Clinical Chemistry 2001; 47: A194.
26) Roos W, Eymann E, Symannek M, et al. Monoclonal antibodies to human heart fatty acid-binding protein. Journal of Immunological Methods 1995; 183: 149-153.
27) Watanabe T, Ohkubo Y, Matsuoka H, et al. Development of a simple whole blood panel test for detection of human heart-type fatty acid-binding protein. Clinical Biochemistry 2001; 34: 257-263.

28) van der Voort D, McNeil CA, Renneberg R, Korf J, Hermens WT, Glatz JFC. Biosensors: basic features and application for fatty acid-binding protein, an early plasma marker of myocardial injury. Sensors and Actuators 2005; 105: 50-59.
29) Pelsers MMAL, Chapelle J-P, Knapen M, *et al.* Influence of age and sex and day-to-day and within-day biological variation on plasma concentrations of fatty acid-binding protein and myoglobin in healthy subjects. Clinical Chemistry 1999; 45: 441-443.
30) Pagani F, Bonara R, Bonetti G, Panteghini M. Evaluation of a sandwich enzyme-linked immunosorbent assay for the measurement of serum fatty acid-binding protein. Annals of Clinical Biochemistry 2002; 39: 404-405.
31) Tsuji R, Tanaka T, Sohmiya K, *et al.* Human heart-type cytoplasmic fatty acid-binding protein in serum and urine during hyperacute myocardial infarction. International Journal of Cardiology 1993; 41: 209-217.
32) Górski J, Hermens WT, Borawski J, Mysliwiec M, Glatz JFC. Increased fatty acid-binding protein concentration in plasma of patients with chronic renal failure. Clinical Chemistry 1997; 43: 193-195.
33) Glatz JF, van Bilsen M, Paulussen RJ, Veerkamp JH, van der Vusse GJ, Reneman RS. Release of fatty acid-binding protein from isolated rat heart subjected to ischemia and reperfusion or to the calcium paradox. Biochimica et Biophysica Acta 1998; 961: 148-152.
34) Okamoto F, Sohmiya K, Ohkaru Y, *et al.* Human heart-type cytoplasmic fatty acid-binding protein (H-FABP) for the diagnosis of acute myocardial infarction. Clinical evaluation of H-FABP in comparison with myoglobin and creatine kinase isoenzyme MB. Clinical Chemistry and Laboratory Medicine 2000; 38: 231-238.
35) Glatz JFC, Haastrup B, Hermens WT, *et al*. Fatty acid-binding protein and the early detection of acute myocardial infarction: the EUROCARDI multicenter trial. Circulation 1997; 96: SuppI I-215.
36) Kleine AH, Glatz JFC, Van Nieuwenhoven FA, Van der Vusse GJ. Release of heart fatty acid-binding protein into plasma after acute myocardial infarction. Molecular and Cellular Biochemistry 1992; 116: 155-162.
37) Chan CPY, Sanderson JE, Glatz JFC, Cheng WS, Hempel A, Renneberg R. A superior early myocardial infarction marker. Human heart-type fatty acid-binding protein. Zeitschrift für Kardiologie 2004; 93: 388-397.
38) Wodzig KWH, Kragten JA, Modrzejewski W, *et al.* Thrombolytic therapy does not change the release ratios of enzymatic and non-

enzymatic myocardial marker proteins. Clinica Chimica Acta 1998; 272: 209-223.
39) Ishii J, Wang J-H, Naruse H, et al. Serum concentrations of myoglobin vs human heart- type cytoplasmic fatty acid-binding protein in early detection of acute myocardial infarction. Clinical. Chemistry 1997; 43: 1372-1378.
40) Sorichter S, Mair J, Koller A, Pelsers MM, Puschendorf B, Glatz JF. Early assessment of exercise induced skeletal muscle injury using plasma fatty acid binding protein. British Journal of Sports Medicine 1998; 32: 121-124.
41) Pelsers, MM, Hermens, WT, Glatz JF. Fatty acid-binding proteins as plasma markers of tissue injury. Clinica Chimica Acta 2005; 352: 15-35.
42) Katrukha A, Bereznekiva A, Filatov V, et al. Improved detection of minor ischemic cardiac injury in patients with unstable angina by measurement of cTnI and Fatty Acid Binding Protein (H-FABP). Clinical Chemistry 1999; 45: A139.
43) Koga H, Saito T, Oshima S, et al. The human heart type fatty acid binding protein is an early biochemical marker in patients with unstable angina pectoris. Circulation 2000; 102: Suppl II-520.
44) Tambara K, Fujita M, Miyamoto S, Doi K, Nishimura K, Komeda M. Pericardial fluid level of heart-type cytoplasmic fatty acid-binding protein (H-FABP) is an indicator of severe myocardial ischemia. International Journal of Cardiology 2004; 93: 281-284.
45) Ghani F, Wu AHB, Graff L, et al. Role of heart-type fatty acid-binding protein in early detection of acute myocardial infarction. Clinical Chemistry.2000; 46, 718-719.
46) Alansari SE, Croal BL. Diagnostic value of heart fatty acid binding protein and myoglobin in patients admitted with chest pain. Annals Clinical Biochemistry 2004; 41: 391-396.
47) Haastrup B, Gill S, Kristensen SR, et al. Biochemical markers of ischaemia for the early identification of acute myocardial infarction without ST segment elevation. Cardiology 2002; 94: 254-261.
48) Braunwald E. Myocardial reperfusion, limitation of infarct size, reduction of left ventricular dysfunction, and improved survival. Should the paradigm be expanded? Circulation 1989; 79: 441-444.
49) Glatz JFC, Kleine AH, van Nieuwenhoven FA., Hermens WT, van Dieijen-Visser MP, van der Vusse GJ. Fatty-acid-binding protein as a plasma marker for the estimation of myocardial infarct size in humans. British Heart Journal 1994; 71: 135-140.
50) Wodzig KWH, Kragten JA, Hermens WT, Glatz JFC, van Dieijen-Visser P. Estimation of myocardial infarct size from

plasma myoglobin or fatty acid-binding protein. Influence of renal function. European Journal of Clinical Chemistry and Clinical Biochemistry 1997; 35: 191-198.

51) de Groot MJ, Wodzig KW, Simoons ML, Glatz JF, Hermens WT. Measurement of myocardial infarct size from plasma fatty acid-binding protein or myoglobin, using individually estimated clearance rates. Cardiovascular Research 1999; 44: 315-324.

52) Ishii J, Nagamura Y, Nomura M, *et al.* Early detection of successful coronary reperfusion based on serum concentration of human heart-type cytoplasmic fatty acid-binding protein. Clinica Chimica Acta. 1997; 262: 13-27.

53) de Lemos JA, Antman EM, Morrow DA, *et al.* Heart-type fatty acid binding protein as a marker of reperfusion after thrombolytic therapy. Clinica Chimica Acta. 2000; 298: 85-97.

54) Abe S, Okino H, Lee S, *et al.* Human heart fatty acid-binding protein, a sensitive and specific marker of coronary reperfusion. Circulation 1991; 84: Suppl II-291.

55) Setsuta K, Seino Y, Takahashi N, *et al.* Clinical significance of elevated levels of cardiac troponin T in patients with chronic heart failure. American Journal of Cardiology 1999; 84, 608-611.

56) Missov E, Mair J. A novel biochemical approach to congestive heart failure: cardiac troponin T. American Heart Journal 1991; 138: 95-99.

57) Chen YN, Wei JR, Zeng LJ, Wu MY. Monitoring of cardiac troponin I in patients with acute heart failure. Annals of Clinical Biochemistry 1999; 36: 433-437.

58) Setsuta K, Seino Y, Ogawa T, Arao M, Miyatake Y, Takano T. Use of cytosolic and myofibril markers in the detection of ongoing myocardial damage in patients with chronic heart failure. American Journal of Medicine 2002; 113: 717-722.

59) Arimoto T, Takeishi Y, Shiga R, *et al.* Prognostic value of elevated circulating heart-type fatty acid binding protein in patients with congestive heart failure. Journal of Cardiac Failure 2005; 11: 56-60.

60) Nakata T, Hashimoto A, Hase M, Tsuchihashi K, Shimamoto K. Human heart-type fatty acid-binding protein as an early diagnostic and prognostic marker in acute coronary syndrome. Cardiology 2003; 99: 96-104.

61) Ishii J, Ozaki Y, Lu J, Kitagawa F, *et al.* Prognostic value of serum concentration of heart-type fatty acid-binding protein relative to cardiac troponin T on admission in the early hours of acute coronary syndrome. Clinical Chemistry 2005; 51: 1397-1404.

62) Takeda S, Kashiwagi H, Kajiwara H, *et al.* Prognostic value of heart fatty acid binding protein for chest symptom patients in emergency room. Circulation 2003; 108 Suppl IV: 582.
63) Erlikh A, Trifonov I, Katrukha A, Gratsiansky N. Prognostic value of serum heart fatty acid-binding protein in patients with non-ST elevation acute coronary syndrome: results of follow-up for 6 months. Circulation 2003; 108: Suppl IV 648.

6: Evidence based review in Neurosciences: Management of Head Injury

DR STEPHEN WILSON, DR PAUL MURPHY and PROF MARK BELLAMY

Introduction
Traumatic brain injury is reaching almost epidemic proportions in the developing world and is recognised as one of the most devastating and potentially life altering conditions in medicine. Overall severe traumatic head injury represents an enormous socioeconomic burden on society with an estimated cost in the European Union of €1200 to €7500 per patient. Over 750 000 patients present with head injury to emergency departments every year equating to a potential cost in excess of €3 billion annually throughout Europe. In the UK Department of Health's third annual report in 2001 focusing on rehabilitation following head injury, over 1 million people per year were estimated to present to UK Accident and Emergency Departments and of these over 100 000 will have moderate to severe injuries [1-3]. The majority of head injured patients in the UK are under 35 years old and 75% are male. The primary mechanism of head injuries is road traffic accidents and with cars becoming faster and roads becoming increasingly congested these statistics are unlikely to fall in the future. Up to 40% of head injuries will also involve alcohol consumption.

Despite this relatively high prevalence and the huge costs to society, there is a distinct lack of large randomised controlled trials to guide patient management. A consensus approach to traumatic brain injury management has been tried and there are now two guideline documents available. One was published in 1997 by the European Brain Injury Consortium (EBIC) [4], the other in 2000 by the American Brain Injury Consortium (ABIC) in collaboration with the Brain Trauma Foundation (BTF) [5].

The European Brain Injury Consortium was founded in 1994 with the aim of "developing a strong clinical group to advise and to work in partnership with sponsors in order to ensure excellence in the design, conduct and analysis of clinical trials in head injury". Their guideline document drew heavily on expert opinion as they recognised the lack of high quality evidence for the majority of interventions used in head injury management. They also recognised that, despite this, clinicians treating brain injured patients would value guidance. The result was a fairly brief, quite readable, pragmatic approach to traumatic brain injury with the majority of the recommendations being based on expert opinion.

In contrast, the Brain Trauma Foundation and the American Association of Neurological Surgeons attempted to produce a set of standards that could be supported by an evidence base. The resulting document, a cumbersome 286 pages, could only support four definitive standards of care that all describe what should not be done rather than what should. There were a further seven recommendations based on 'level 2 evidence'.

It would appear that traumatic brain injury received very little input from clinical researchers and yet this is not the case; a working party chaired by Narayan in 2002 [6] concluded that there were over 250 clinical trials either published or ongoing examining various aspects of traumatic brain injury management. Unfortunately the quality of many of the trials is poor. The Cochrane Collaboration have also been active in investigating aspects of traumatic brain injury management and so far there have been 15 systematic reviews performed on topics ranging from specialist interventional therapies such as excitatory amino acids and noradrenergic agonists to mainstream therapies such as barbiturates and therapeutic hypothermia. There are a further three Cochrane reviews that are currently at the protocol stage. Once again, the problem faced by the reviewers has been that of limited evidence with two reviews unable to identify a single trial that met inclusion criteria. Of the remaining 13 reviews, nine highlighted the other significant problem in the management of severe head injury, that of lack of efficacy. Very few interventions in head injury management have proven to be of undeniable benefit in terms of improved outcome. Only three Cochrane systematic reviews concluded that some therapies were beneficial. The final review of corticosteroids for acute traumatic brain injury [7] was heavily influenced by the MRC CRASH study [8] and concluded that steroids were detrimental in traumatic brain injury. All this may go some way to explaining why there has been no significant improvement in patient outcomes from traumatic brain injury in the past 10 years [9].

The aim of this review is to summarise and condense the relevant issues from the European Brain Injury Consortium and Brain Trauma Foundation guidelines, the Cochrane Collaboration reports and the other independent reviewers whilst also providing some simple answers to clinical questions about treating the severely brain injured patient such as:

MANAGEMENT OF HEAD INJURY

- Where should traumatic brain injury be managed? In the neurointensive care unit (ICU) or the district general hospital?
- How do we monitor patients with traumatic brain injury – intracranial pressure (ICP) or cerebral perfusion pressure (CPP) targeted therapy and which intracranial pressure monitor is best?
- Should we cool patients with traumatic brain injury?
- Should we hyperventilate patients with traumatic brain injury?
- What are the roles for barbiturate coma and decompressive craniectomy?
- Is there a need for more invasive and more complex monitoring?
- What is the role for mannitol and hypertonic saline?
- Who should be fed and when?
- Does protocol led management improve outcome in traumatic brain injury?

Methods

While this is not a systematic review, Medline and Embase databases were searched using the terms: head injury and traumatic brain injury and management linked with the Boolean operator 'AND'. The search was refined by limiting the results to human, adult, English language articles. Other review articles were isolated and cross-referenced. The Cochrane Database of Systematic Reviews for articles relating to head injury or brain injury was also searched.

The National Clinical Trials Database (http://www.clinicaltrials.gov) was reviewed for ongoing research into head injury as was the web site of the National Institute for Clinical and Healthcare Excellence (NICE) (http://www.nice.org.uk).

Where should patients with traumatic brain injuries be managed?

It has been estimated that up to 40% of severely brain injured patients are managed in non-neurosurgical centres in the UK. These centres will, in general, have limited facilities for invasive intracranial pressure monitoring and as such any protocol for management based upon maintenance of an adequate cerebral perfusion pressure will be impossible, despite some evidence that this may be beneficial in non-surgical lesions [10, 11]. Added to this, there is no facility for subsequent surgical intervention if this becomes necessary without referral to a neurosurgeon. The reasons for continued management in non-neurosurgical centres are unclear. It may be that patients managed in non-neurosurgical centres are deemed to be unsalvageable at the time of presentation. However, neurosurgeons may be loathe to accept patients who do not require immediate surgical intervention due to limited resources and so quite rightly ration the available neurosurgical beds to treat those patients who do need immediate surgery.

The recently published article by Patel et al. [9] is one of the few studies in head injury management providing level 1 evidence. In a prospective observational study of 176 447 patients entered into the Trauma Audit and Research Database between 1989 and 2003, they identified 22 216 (13%) as having a head injury, of whom 6921 had abbreviated injury scale (AIS) scores above 2 (representing a severe brain injury). The authors' first point was that there appeared to have been an overall reduction in the risk of death from head injury by 1.5% per year since 1989. However, closer examination of the results showed that almost the entire reduction had occurred between 1989 and 1994 and there had been no significant reduction in the risk of death in the following nine years.

Comparison between the patients presenting with head injury and those with non-head injury trauma emphasised the socioeconomic burden and demographic distribution of traumatic brain injury; the median age of head injury patients was below 35 while that of the non-head injured population was 43 years. Head injured patients were also on average more severely injured with median injury severity scores of 20-25 compared with 9 in the non-head injured group. The most striking difference, however, was the incidence of death which was over 7 times greater in the head injured population (25-31% versus 3%).

The authors then analysed 6921 severely injured patients in greater detail by dividing them into 4616 (66%) managed in a neurosurgical centre and 2305 (34%) managed in a non-neurosurgical centre. Those managed in the neurosurgical centre were slightly younger and were more likely to have had an isolated head injury (44% versus 39%). Injury severity scores and admission Glasgow Coma Scale (GCS) scores were the same for both groups. The mortality for patients treated in a neurosurgical centre was 35% while for those treated in a non-neurosurgical centre it was 61%. It has been estimated that if these figures are correct, then in the 8 years of the study 2000 lives could have been saved if all severe head injury patients had been managed in neurosurgical units.

In their discussion, the authors acknowledge a number of limitations in their study. For example, the observational approach may have led to case selection bias. However, they felt that to obtain the same level of evidence by recruiting and randomising 6000 patients to different locations of care would have been logistically impossible. They also acknowledge that patients not transferred may have injuries deemed incompatible with life, or simply did not require neurosurgical intervention. They therefore adjusted their case mix to compensate for this and found that there was still a 2-fold increase in the odds of death for patients treated in a non-neurosurgical unit. If the results are accurate, it could have enormous consequences for regional neurosurgical units.

The underlying message and the current recommended guideline is that all patients with a severe head injury should be managed in a unit with 24 hour neurosurgical facilities [10].

How do we monitor patients with traumatic brain injury – intracranial pressure or cerebral perfusion pressure targeted therapy and which intracranial pressure monitor is best?

There are no level 1 studies demonstrating an improved outcome from either intracranial pressure or cerebral perfusion pressure targeted therapy. However, intracranial pressure monitoring has become a standard of care in head injury management ever since Marmarou *et al*. [12] in the early 1990s showed that patients whose intracranial pressures were persistently greater than 20 mmHg suffered poorer outcomes. In 2001 Struchen *et al*. [13] described poorer outcomes in patients whose cerebral perfusion pressure dropped below 60 mmHg and Chambers *et al*. [14] also demonstrated worse outcomes in patients with cerebral perfusion pressure below 55 mmHg. All these studies were prospective observational studies without blinding or randomisation. It is generally agreed that attempting to perform an outcome study using a control group randomised to not receive intracranial pressure monitoring would almost certainly be unethical. Both the European Brain Injury Consortium and the Brain Trauma Foundation guidelines agree that intracranial pressure monitoring is unequivocally indicated in the patient with severe head injury and an abnormal CT scan. This is summarised as:

Head Injury + Ventilator + Abnormal CT Scan = ICP Monitor

The exact therapeutic targets that should guide therapy are also contentious. Rosner's group [15] in 1995 advocated therapy targeted towards the maintenance of a 'normal' cerebral perfusion pressure. In their original paper, they described outcomes from 158 patients managed with a protocol aimed at maintaining a cerebral perfusion pressure above 70 mmHg. The overall mortality was 29%, with good neurological outcomes in 59% of the patients. These data appeared to compare favourably with the prospective observational data on almost

750 patients recorded in the Traumatic Coma Data Bank (TCDB) for whom 35% mortality was predicted [16].

In 1999, Robertson et al. [17] described a randomised controlled trial of 189 patients treated with either a cerebral perfusion pressure targeted protocol (cerebral perfusion pressure >70 mmHg) or an intracranial pressure targeted protocol (intracranial pressure <20 mmHg). The group treated with cerebral perfusion pressure targeted therapy had significantly higher mean arterial pressures, cerebral perfusion pressures, end tidal CO_2 and cerebral blood flows (CBF) than the intracranial pressure targeted group. They also report a significant reduction in the incidence of jugular venous bulb desaturation (their primary outcome) from 50.6% to 30%. Cerebral perfusion pressure targeted therapy has become the treatment standard in the majority of centres. This is supported by both the European Brain Injury Consortium and the Brain Trauma Foundation guidelines. However, the level above which cerebral perfusion pressure should be maintained is again contentious: 60 mmHg seems to be the standard despite there being no randomised controlled trial data to support this variable. This provides a pragmatic compromise between the levels used by Robertson [17] (i.e. >70 mmHg) which, although improving cerebral outcomes, produced a 5-fold increase in the incidence of respiratory complications and pressures advocated by Eker et al. [18] (see below).

Forsyth et al. [19] for the Cochrane group performed a systematic review of routine intracranial pressure monitoring in acute coma. Their primary objective was to identify whether intracranial pressure monitoring reduced the risk of death or severe disability in all cases of severe coma. They identified 11 studies involving intracranial pressure monitoring but ultimately excluded them all from the proposed meta-analysis and as such concluded that there are no data from randomised controlled trials that could clarify the role of intracranial pressure monitoring in acute coma. The reasons for excluding the trials included non-randomisation in six trials and randomisation to different treatment groups in the other trials.

A further strategy for traumatic brain injury management was described by Eker [18] and colleagues from Lund University Hospital, Sweden. Their approach targets cerebral tissue perfusion and blood volume regulation in the presence of a disrupted blood brain barrier and loss of cerebral autoregulatory function. This approach differs quite markedly from the intracranial pressure / cerebral perfusion pressure targeted therapies. In a non-randomised, prospective study of 53 patients treated with the 'Lund protocol' compared with 38 historical controls treated with a cerebral perfusion pressure targeted strategy the mortality in the treatment group was only 8% compared with 47% in the control group. There was no significant difference in the proportions of patients with severe disability. These data appear promising but the study suffers from a number of significant limitations. First it is very small with only 53 patients in the treatment group. Second the use of historical controls introduces a number of potential sources of bias such as patient entry timing, nurse and doctor involvement, differing qualities of intensive care management and changes in other aspects of care over time. Third it is interesting to note that the baseline mortality for the control group was 47% which is markedly greater than the 35% mortality for a similar patient population treated in neurosurgical centres in the UK [9]. This further highlights the limitations of using historical control groups. The authors accept many of these limitations in their discussion and the overriding message is that a large randomised controlled trial is needed to clarify this issue.

At present the best evidence suggests that cerebral perfusion pressure targeted therapy is to be preferred and the cerebral perfusion pressure should be maintained above 60 mmHg [4].

The choice of intracranial pressure monitor is often left to individual centre's expertise and available resources. There is very little data to support any single method in preference over another. The two most commonly employed methods are intraventricular fluid filled ventriculostomies and intraparenchymal fibreoptic devices. The 2000 Brain Trauma Foundation guidelines ranked the various methods available based on a risk-benefit analysis and put ventriculostomies above intraparenchymal devices. Ventriculostomies represent a standard of care in the USA where they are also used therapeutically. In the UK and Europe, fibreoptic devices are more common with cerebrospinal fluid drainage forming only a later part of management. The risks for both methods include infection, bleeding, cerebrospinal fluid leak and seizures. In their literature review, the authors of the Brain Trauma Foundation guidelines identified a colonisation risk of 5% for ventriculostomies and 14% for intraparenchymal devices. Bleeding was similar for both methods. Malfunction rates were between 9 and 40% for fibreoptic devices but only 6.3% for ventriculostomies [21-24]. The commonest cause of malfunction in fibreoptic devices is zero-line drift. This is not a problem with fluid filled devices as they can be re-zeroed regularly. The recorded drift can be quite marked, up to 4 mmHg in the first 24 hours [24] and up to 3.3 mmHg per day over 5 days [25]. It was noted, however, that ventriculostomies may be more difficult to insert, especially in the patient with raised intracranial pressure and cerebral swelling with marked reduction in ventricular volume.

On balance it would seem that ventriculostomies may represent a better approach to intracranial pressure monitoring than intraparenchymal fibreoptic devices [20].

Should we cool patients with traumatic brain injury?
This is one of the few areas of traumatic brain injury management where level 1 evidence exists. Alderson and colleagues for the Cochrane group performed a systematic review of therapeutic hypothermia in 2004 [26]. The group identified 14 trials with a total with 1094 subjects. Their overall conclusion was that "there is no evidence that hypothermia is beneficial in the treatment of head injury". Therapeutic hypothermia was associated with an odds ratio for death alone of 0.8 (95% confidence interval (CI) 0.61 to 1.04) and an odds ratio for death or severe disability of 0.75 (95% CI 0.56 to 1.00). The authors also commented that the odds ratio for developing pneumonia was significantly increased at 1.95 (95% CI 1.18 to 3.23). The reasons for this failure of hypothermia may be related to the timing of intervention. Rapid rewarming may be harmful and a subgroup analysis [27] of data taken from the NABIS:H (National Acute Brain Injury Study: Hypothermia) trial [28] suggested that of the 28% of patients with admission temperatures below 35°C randomised to normothermia, 78% died or were severely disabled. Of the remaining group, there appeared to be a trend towards improved outcome. Patients aged over 45 years had worse outcomes with hypothermia. From their work, they have suggested that patients hypothermic on admission who are under 45 years old may benefit from hypothermia and as a result a second trial NABIS:H II is being performed to specifically to investigate this.

The European Brain Injury Consortium guidelines also do not support the routine use of therapeutic hypothermia stating that as an unproven form of intracranial pressure therapy, it should not be used in patients enrolled into clinical trials of other intracranial pressure therapies as the potential interactions would be unpredictable.

Should we hyperventilate patients with traumatic brain injury?
Hyperventilation has been used to control intractable elevated intracranial pressure for more than 20 years since Gordon [29] described better neurological outcomes in ventilated patients following traumatic coma. The effects of hyperventilation, however, are only transient with the cerebral arterioles returning to their original calibre within 4 to 6 hrs and hence the effective reduction in cerebral

blood flow is negated [30]. The only randomised controlled trial of hyperventilation in head injury was performed by Muizelaar [31] in 1991. The 77 patients who were hyperventilated for 5 days to a PaCO$_2$ of 25 mmHg (3.2kPa) had poorer outcomes at 3 and 6 months. One mechanism for this deleterious effect may be reduced cerebral blood flow and resulting cerebral ischaemia secondary to intense cerebral vasoconstriction. Studies using Xenon enhanced CT and positron emission tomography (PET) imaging have measured cerebral blood flows of less than 20 ml/100g/min (compared to a normal value of 50 ml/100g/min). The effects of hyperventilation on the injured brain are unreliable in the absence of the normal autoregulatory mechanisms with some patients developing relative oligaemia whilst others become hyperaemic [32,33]. There is also evidence that regional variation in cerebral blood flow may contribute to the unpredictable effects of hyperventilation.

A Cochrane review by Roberts and Schierhout [34] in 1997 identified three trials of hyperventilation but only Muizelaar's [31] could be included. As such no recommendation could be made as to the relative benefits or harmful effects of hyperventilation. The European Brain Injury Consortium guidelines recommend that hyperventilation to a PaCO$_2$ below 4 kPa should only be undertaken as a temporising measure whilst other methods of intracranial pressure control are attempted [4]. They also recommend alternative methods of monitoring cerebral oxygenation such as jugular bulb catheters or intracerebral tissue oxygen analysers.

What are the roles for barbiturate coma and decompressive craniectomy?

Barbiturates have been used to control intractable intracranial pressure for many years and there is certainly no doubt that in the majority of patients, the intracranial pressure will fall after a large dose of thiopentone. The mechanisms behind this effect are two fold. Barbiturates reduce the cerebral metabolic requirement for oxygen to 25% of baseline. They also cause a marked reduction in mean arterial pressure in a quarter of patients treated and this in turn will reduce cerebral blood volume and hence intracranial pressure. The effects on cerebral perfusion pressure are more complex. Barbiturates have theoretical effects on calcium flux within the brain and on gamma-aminobutyric acid (GABA) receptors which may be beneficial. Significant side effects, however, include hypotension, sodium accumulation and unreactive pupils making further patient assessment difficult. There is also the prolonged recovery time which can make accurate assessment of brain stem death difficult.

A Cochrane review of five randomised and quasi-randomised trials by Roberts [35] in 2000 could find "no evidence that barbiturate therapy in patients with acute severe head injury improves outcome". They also noted that 1 in 4 patients will have a fall in mean arterial pressure which will offset any beneficial effects on cerebral perfusion pressure gained from the reduction in intracranial pressure [36,37].

At the moment, the benefit of decompressive craniectomy is being assessed with two large randomised controlled trials in adults: the Australasian DECRA (Early Decompressive Craniectomy in Patients With Severe Traumatic Brain Injury) Trial [38] and the European and North American RESCUEicp (Randomised Evaluation of Surgery with Craniectomy for Uncontrollable Elevation of Intra-Cranial Pressure) Study [39]. In 2006, the Cochrane group reviewed the efficacy of secondary decompressive craniectomy on outcome and quality of life in patients with severe traumatic brain injury with refractory raised intracranial pressure [40]. Only one paper by Taylor *et al.* [41] met the inclusion criteria. In a prospective randomised controlled trial, they assessed the effect of secondary decompression on death and disability in 27 children. The relative risks of death and unfavourable outcome in the treated group were lower than in the untreated group (relative risk = 0.54 for both (95% CI for death 0.17 to 1.72; 95% CI for death, severe disability or vegetative state 0.29 to 1.07)). There were no trials identified by the Cochrane group in adult patients. The Cochrane report stated that "there is no evidence to support the routine use of secondary decompressive craniectomy to reduce unfavourable outcome in adults with severe traumatic brain injury and refractory high ICP". They also commented that the only trial in children, although small, did suggest that secondary decompressive craniectomy may be beneficial in patients under 18 years old in whom maximal medical therapy had failed to control refractory raised intracranial pressures. Further non-randomised and quasi-randomised controlled trial data has supported the case for secondary decompressive craniectomy. Both the DECRA and RESCUEicp trials are designed to address this question.

Is there a need for more invasive and more complex monitoring?
Advances in medical technology have introduced a raft of ancillary monitoring devices for brain injured patients and with the current vogue for goal directed therapies [42-44], it is tempting to think that one may prove useful in improving outcome from severe traumatic brain injury.

Transcranial Doppler is a potentially useful non-invasive tool, used quite extensively in the management of subarachnoid haemorrhage to assess vasospasm; it has similar uses in traumatic brain injury [45, 46]. It can only provide a global assessment of large vessel blood velocity and provides no real indication of microvascular tone or regional variations in flow dynamics. Problems with bony interference can limit its use. It can, however, usefully distinguish between a high intracranial pressure in relation to low cerebral perfusion pressure and a high intracranial pressure in relation to hyperaemia. It can also be used to test for a pressure passive circulation where autoregulation has been impaired.

Jugular bulb venous saturation measures the oxygen content in the venous effluent from the brain using a retrograde internal jugular catheter. It provides a global assessment of oxygen uptake by brain tissue and can also be used to calculate cerebral blood flow from the arterio-venous difference. Observational studies have described a correlation between poor outcomes from traumatic brain injury and jugular bulb desaturation or low arterio-jugular oxygen difference ($AJDO_2$) [47-50].

Near infrared spectroscopy (NIRS) is primarily a research tool, not commonly used in clinical setting. Again it provides global averages for oxygen content.

Cerebral microdialysis is another research tool although it is slowly entering clinical practice in some centres. Microdialysis can be used to measure various markers of anaerobic metabolism and cell membrane disruption in local brain tissue including glucose, glutamate, lactate, pyruvate and the lactate/pyruvate ratio. Results will depend on catheter position and there is no consensus view on the correct site.

Cerebral tissue oxygen / CO2 content is being investigated as it provides localised results for brain tissue oxygen and CO_2 levels.

Multimodal monitoring involves a combination of intraparenchymal monitoring modalities, microdialysis, brain tissue oxygenation and intracranial pressure monitoring. This is a research tool and is not widely available.

Clinical evidence for the benefit of all these techniques is extremely limited and there are no outcome studies of any in traumatic brain injury. It is, however, recommended by both the European Brain Injury Consortium and Brain Trauma Foundation guidelines that "aggressive hyperventilation…may be employed provided monitoring of cerebral oxygenation is instituted, usually with a jugular bulb catheter" [4].

What is the role for mannitol and hypertonic saline?

Mannitol is commonly used to control raised intracranial pressure in the head injured patient. A survey by Jeevaratnam [51] in 1996 concluded that 100% of UK neurosurgical centres used mannitol in the treatment of raised intracranial pressure. A Cochrane review by Wakai et al. [52] in 2005 identified seven trials involving the comparison of mannitol with different doses of mannitol, placebo standard care or other intracranial pressure lowering therapies. Five hundred and sixty patients were included overall. The authors' concluded that "high dose mannitol (1.2-1.4 g/kg) may be preferable to conventional-dose mannitol in the acute management of comatose patients with severe head injury". This was based on three studies by Cruz and colleagues comparing doses of mannitol between 1.2 to 1.4 g/kg with doses of 0.6 to 0.7 g/kg [53-55] which showed a relative risk of death of 0.56 (95% CI 0.39 to 0.79) and relative risk of death or severe disability at 6 months of 0.58 (95% CI 0.47 to 0.72). Intracranial pressure directed therapy appeared to show a marginal benefit over therapy based on clinical and physiological signs (relative risk =0.83, 95% CI 0.47 to 1.46) [56].

One paper also compared 20% mannitol 2 ml/kg with 7.5% hypertonic saline 2 ml/kg [57], showing a relative risk for death of 1.25 (95% CI 0.47 to 3.33) in favour of the hypertonic saline group. The Cochrane authors concluded that "mannitol may have a detrimental effect when compared to hypertonic saline", however, the study was very small (n=20) and the 95% CI extremely wide (0.47-3.33). Further studies investigating the role of hypertonic saline with and without dextran are planned including a large, multi-centre study of over 2000 patients in North America investigating pre-hospital administration of hypertonic saline to traumatic brain injury patients [58].

The European Brain Injury Consortium guidelines recommend "infusion of 0.25 to 0.5 g/kg 20% mannitol over 15 to 20 minutes, repeated as necessary with frequent measurement of blood osmolarity and maintenance of serum osmolarity below 315 mosm/kg". This would appear to contradict the findings of the Cochrane group in respect of the dose of mannitol. However the high dose group received mannitol prior to the insertion of intracranial pressure monitoring and were treated on the basis of pupillary reactions [54] or CT scan findings of acute sub-dural haematoma [53]. No study has adequately assessed the use of mannitol to reduce elevated intracranial pressure in terms of outcome and further large randomised controlled trials are needed to clarify this issue.

Who should be fed and when?
Yanagawa *et al.* [59] for the Cochrane group performed a systematic review of nutritional support in head injured patients. Eleven studies were included involving 534 patients. Seven trials assessed the timing of nutritional support and seven assessed the route (parenteral versus enteral). The conclusions from their meta-analysis were that the relative risk of death with early nutrition (within 72 hrs) was 0.67 (95% CI: 0.41-1.07) and the risk for death or severe disability 0.75 (95% CI: 0.5-1.11). In analysing the route of administration the authors found the relative risk for death to be 0.66 (95% CI: 0.41-1.07) in favour of parenteral nutrition. They note, however, that in three of the trials nasogastric feeding was used early and that the observed results may have been related to the timing of the intervention rather than the route.

The Brain Trauma Foundation guidelines state that "nutritional support should be provided using enteral or parenteral formulas...by day 7 after injury". The Cochrane group conclude that "early feeding may be associated with a trend towards better outcomes in terms of survival and disability". The European Brain Injury Consortium guidelines advocate "early institution of enteral feeding". All the groups who have investigated this issue recommend that further randomised controlled trials are required.

Conclusions
Good quality evidence is lacking for most aspects of traumatic brain injury management. This has been highlighted by the Brain Trauma Foundation guidelines [5] which could only recommend three standards of care: avoidance of chronic prolonged hyperventilation, avoidance of steroids specifically to treat head injury and avoidance of prophylactic anticonvulsants to prevent late post-traumatic epilepsy. The European Brain Injury Consortium guidelines [4] fare no better with many of their recommendations being based upon low-level trial evidence and expert opinion. Both these guideline documents do however provide useful background for developing treatment protocols that can guide trainee intensivists and also provide a template for comparable research in the future. More large randomised controlled trials are needed to clarify the contentious issues in head injury management and also to improve patient care and ultimately restore the gradual improvements in mortality that were seen in the early 1990s.

Post Script
There are ten further Cochrane reviews that have not been discussed in this chapter for the sake of brevity. Of these, the only two with definitive conclusions were Schierhout and Roberts paper from 2001 [60] stating that "there is no evidence that treatment with prophylactic anti-epileptics reduces the occurrence of late seizures, or has any effect on death and neurological disability"; and Alderson and Roberts from 2005 [7] who concluded that "the increase in mortality with steroids [in the MRC-CRASH Trial [8]] suggest that steroids should no longer be routinely used in people with traumatic head injury".

References
1. United Kingdom Parliament. Select Committee on Health. Third Annual Report. Head Injury: Rehabilitation. London: The Stationery Office by Order of the House. 28 March 2001. http://www.parliament.uk/commons/hsecom.htm.
2. The British Society of Rehabilitation Medicine. Rehabilitation after traumatic brain injury. London: British Society of Rehabilitation Medicine, 1998. pp 9-10.
3. Teasdale G, Murray G, Parker L, Jennett B. Adding up the Glasgow Coma Score. Acta Neurochirurgica (Wien) 1979; 28: 13-16.
4. Maas AIR, Dearden M, Teasdale GM, et al. EBIC-Guidelines for Management of Severe Head Injury in Adults. Acta Neurochirurgica (Wien) 1997; 139: 286-294.
5. Bullock M, Chesnut R, Clifton G, et al. Management and Prognosis of Severe Traumatic Brain Injury: a joint project of The Brain Trauma Foundation and The American Association of Neurological Surgeons, Joint Section on Neurotrauma and Critical Care. New York: Brain Trauma Foundation, 2000. http://www2.braintrauma.org/guidelines/index.php.
6. Narayan R, Michel M, Ansell B. Clinical Trials in Head Injury. Journal of Neurotrauma 2002; 19: 503-557.
7. Alderson P, Roberts I. Corticosteroids for acute traumatic brain injury. Cochrane Database of Systematic Reviews 2005; 1.
8. Roberts I, Yates D, Sandercock P, et al. Effect of intravenous corticosteroids on death within 14 days in 10008 adults with clinically significant head injury (MRC CRASH trial): randomised placebo-controlled trial. Lancet 2004; 364: 1321-1328.
9. Patel H, Bouamra O, Woodford M, King A, Yates D, Lecky F. Trends in head injury outcome from 1989 to 2003 and the effect of neurosurgical care: an observational study. Lancet 2005; 366: 1538-1544.

10. Patel H, Menon D, Tebbs S, Hawker R, Hutchinson P, Kirkpatrick P. Specialist neurocritical care and outcome from head injury. Intensive Care Medicine 2002; 28: 547-553.
11. Stocchetti N, Rossi S, Buzzi F, Mattioli C, Paparella A, Colombo A. Intracranial hypertension in head injury: management and results. Intensive Care Medicine 1999; 25: 371-376.
12. Marmarou A, Anderson R, Ward J, et al. Impact of ICP instability and hypotension on outcome in patients with severe head injury. Journal of Neurosurgery 1991; 75: S59–S64.
13. Struchen M, Hannay H, Contant C, Robertson C. The relation between acute physiological variables and outcome on the Glasgow Outcome Scale and Disability Rating Scale following severe traumatic brain injury. Journal of Neurotrauma 2001; 18: 115-125.
14. Chambers I, Treadwell L, Mendellow A. Determination of threshold levels of cerebral perfusion pressure and intracranial pressure in severe head injury by using receiver-operating characteristic curves: an observational study in 291 patients. Journal of Neurosurgery 2001; 94: 412-416.
15. Rosner M, Rosner S, Johnson A. Cerebral perfusion pressure: management protocol and clinical results. Journal of Neurosurgery 1995; 83: 949-962.
16. Marshall L, Gautille T, Klauber M, et al. The outcome of severe closed head injury. Journal of Neurosurgery 1991; 75: S28-S36.
17. Robertson C, Valadka A, Hannay H, et al. Prevention of secondary ischemic insults after severe head injury. Critical Care Medicine 1999; 27: 2086-2095.
18. Eker C, Asgeirsson B, Grande P, Schalen W, Nordstrom C. Improved outcome after severe head injury with a new therapy based on principles for brain volume regulation and preserved microcirculation. Critical Care Medicine 1998; 26: 1881-1886.
19. Forsyth R, Baxter P, Elliott T. Routine intracranial pressure monitoring in acute coma. Cochrane Database of Systematic Reviews. 2001; 3.
20. Brain Trauma Foundation. The American Association of Neurological Surgeons. The Joint Section on Neurotrauma and Critical Care. Recommendations for intracranial pressure monitoring technology. Journal of Neurotrauma 2000; 17: 497-506.
21. North B, Reilly P. Comparison among three methods of intracranial pressure recording. Neurosurgery 1986; 18: 730-732.
22. Ostrup R, Luerssen T, Marshall L, Zornow M. Continuous monitoring of intracranial pressure with a miniaturized fiberoptic device. Journal of Neurosurgery 1987; 67: 206-209.

23. Bavetta S, Sutcliffe J, Sparrow O, Hamlyn P. A prospective comparison of fibre-optic and fluid-filled single lumen bolt subdural pressure transducers in ventilated neurosurgical patients. British Journal of Neurosurgery 1996; 10: 279-84.
24. Piek J, Bock W. Continuous monitoring of cerebral tissue pressure in neurosurgical practice--experiences with 100 patients. Intensive Care Medicine. 1990; 16: 184-188.
25. Bavetta S, Norris J, Wyatt M, Sutcliffe J, Hamlyn P. Prospective study of zero drift in fiberoptic pressure monitors used in clinical practice. Journal of Neurosurgery 1997; 86: 927-930.
26. Alderson P, Gadkary C, Signorini DF. Therapeutic hypothermia for head injury. Cochrane Database of Systematic Reviews 2004; 4.
27. Valadka AB, Andrews BT. Neurotrauma. Evidence-based Answers to Common Questions. New York: Thieme Medical Publishers, 2005.
28. Clifton G, Miller E, Choi S, *et al*. Lack of effect of induction of hypothermia after acute brain injury. New England Journal of Medicine 2001; 344: 556-563.
29. Gordon E. Controlled respiration in the management of patients with traumatic brain injuries. Acta Anaesthesiologica Scandinavica 1971; 15: 193-208.
30. Carmona-Suazo J, Maas A, van den Brink W, van Santbrink H, Steyerberg E, Avezaat C. CO2 reactivity and brain oxygen pressure monitoring in severe head injury. Critical Care Medicine. 2000; 28: 3268-3274.
31. Muizelaar J, Marmarou A, Ward J, *et al*. Adverse effects of prolonged hyperventilation in patients with severe head injury: a randomized clinical trial. Journal of Neurosurgery 1991; 75: 731-739.
32. Stringer W, Hasso A, Thompson J, Hinshaw D, Jordan K. Hyperventilation-induced cerebral ischemia in patients with acute brain lesions: demonstration by xenon-enhanced CT. American Journal of Neuroradiology 1993; 14: 475-484.
33. Marion D, Bouma G. The use of stable xenon-enhanced computed tomographic studies of cerebral blood flow to define changes in cerebral carbon dioxide vasoresponsivity caused by a severe head injury. Neurosurgery 1991; 29: 869-873.
34. Schierhout G, Roberts I. Hyperventilation therapy for acute traumatic brain injury. Cochrane Database of Systematic Reviews 2000; 2.
35. Roberts I. Barbiturates for acute traumatic brain injury. Cochrane Database of Systematic Reviews 2000; 2.
36. Eisenberg H, Frankowski R, Contant C, Marshall L, Walker M. High-dose barbiturate control of elevated intracranial pressure in

patients with severe head injury. Journal of Neurosurgery 1988; 69: 15-23.
37. Ward J, Becker D, Miller J, *et al*. Failure of prophylactic barbiturate coma in the treatment of severe head injury. Journal of Neurosurgery 1985; 62: 383-388.
38. Cooper DJ, Rosenfeld JV, Murray L, *et al*. DECRA, a multi-centre prospective randomised trial of early decompressive craniectomy in patients with severe traumatic brain injury, protocol version 25. 2004.
http://www.clinicaltrials.gov/ct/show/NCT00155987
39. Hutchinson P, Kirkpatrick P, Menon D, *et al*. RESCUEicp: Randomised Evaluation of Surgery with Craniectomy for Uncontrollable Elevation of Intra-Cranial Pressure. Study protocol, MREC Approved June 2003.
http://www.RESCUEicp.com 2003.
40. Sahuquillo J, Arikan F. Decompressive craniectomy for the treatment of refractory high intracranial pressure in traumatic brain injury. Cochrane Database of Systematic Reviews 2006; 1.
41. Taylor A, Butt W, Rosenfeld J, *et al*. A randomized trial of very early decompressive craniectomy in children with traumatic brain injury and sustained intracranial hypertension. Childs Nervous System 2001; 17: 154-62.
42. Pearse R, Dawson D, Fawcett J, Rhodes A, Grounds RM, Bennett ED. Early goal-directed therapy after major surgery reduces complications and duration of hospital stay. A randomised, controlled trial. Critical Care 2005; 9:R687 - R693.
43. Wilson J, Woods I, Fawcett J, *et al*. Reducing the risk of major elective surgery: randomised controlled trial of preoperative optimisation of oxygen delivery. British Medical Journal 1999; 318: 1099 - 1103.
44. Boyd O, Grounds R, Bennett E. A randomized clinical trial of the effect of deliberate perioperative increase of oxygen delivery on mortality in high-risk surgical patients. Journal of the American Medical Association 1993; 270: 2699 - 2707.
45. Martin N, Doberstein C, Zane C, Caron M, Thomas K, Becker D. Posttraumatic cerebral arterial spasm: transcranial Doppler ultrasound, cerebral blood flow, and angiographic findings. Journal of Neurosurgery 1992; 77: 575-583.
46. Lee J, Martin N, Alsina G, *et al*. Hemodynamically significant cerebral vasospasm and outcome after head injury: a prospective study. Journal of Neurosurgery 1997; 87: 221-233.
47. Cormio M, Valadka A, Robertson C. Elevated jugular venous oxygen saturation after severe head injury. Journal of Neurosurgery 1999; 90: 9-15.

48. Macmillan CSA, Andrews PJD, Easton VJ. Increased jugular bulb saturation is associated with poor outcome in traumatic brain injury. Journal of Neurology, Neurosurgery & Psychiatry 2001; 70: 101-104.
49. Gopinath S, Robertson C, Contant C, et al. Jugular venous desaturation and outcome after head injury. Journal of Neurology, Neurosurgery & Psychiatry 1994; 57: 717-723.
50. Cruz J. Relationship between early patterns of cerebral extraction of oxygen and outcome from severe acute traumatic brain swelling: Cerebral ischemia or cerebral viability? Critical Care Medicine 1996; 24: 953-956.
51. Jeevaratnam DR, Menon DK. Survey of intensive care of severely head injured patients in the United Kingdom. British Medical Journal 1996; 312: 944-947.
52. Wakai A, Roberts I, Schierhout G. Mannitol for acute traumatic brain injury. Cochrane Database of Systematic Reviews 2005; 4.
53. Cruz J, Minoja G, Okuchi K. Improving clinical outcomes from acute subdural hematomas with the emergency preoperative administration of high doses of mannitol: A randomized trial. Neurosurgery 2001; 49: 864-871.
54. Cruz J, Minoja G, Okuchi K. Major clinical and physiological benefits of early high doses of mannitol for intraparenchymal temporal lobe hemorrhages with abnormal pupillary widening: A randomized trial. Neurosurgery 2002; 51: 628-638.
55. Cruz J, Minoja G, Okuchi K, Facco E. Successful use of the new high-dose mannitol treatment in patients with Glasgow Coma Scale scores of 3 and bilateral abnormal pupillary widening: a randomized trial. Journal of Neurosurgery 2004; 100: 376-383.
56. Smith HP, Kelly DL Jr, McWhorter JM, et al. Comparison of mannitol regimens in patients with severe head injury undergoing intracranial monitoring. Journal of Neurosurgery 1986; 65: 820-824.
57. Vialet R, Albanese J, Thomachot L, et al. Isovolume hypertonic solutes (sodium chloride or mannitol) in the treatment of refractory posttraumatic intracranial hypertension: 2 ml/kg 7.5% saline is more effective than 2 ml/kg 20% mannitol. Critical Care Medicine 2003; 31: 1683-1687.
58. Weisfeldt M, Hallstrom A, Powell J, et al. Phase 3 Study of Hypertonic Resuscitation Following Traumatic Brain Injury. Clinical trials identifier NCT00316004. http://www.clinicaltrials.gov/ct/gui/show/NCT00316004;jsessionid=6E589B61546AFBA63CB6E1240EB513E4?order=9 2006.
59. Yanagawa T, Bunn F, Roberts I, Wentz R, Pierro A. Nutritional support for head-injured patients. Cochrane Database of Systematic Reviews 2002; 3.

60. Schierhout G, Roberts I. Anti-epileptic drugs for preventing seizures following acute traumatic brain injury. Cochrane Database of Systematic Reviews 2001; 4.

7: Head injury: The Lund Approach

PROF CARL-HENRIK NORDSTRÖM

Introduction
Two apparently incompatible principles for reduction of increased intracranial pressure (ICP) in severe head injuries were presented in 1994-95. According to the principles from the USA, published by Rosner *et al.* [1], reducing dangerous increases in ICP can be obtained by *increasing* in mean arterial blood pressure (MAP) and cerebral perfusion pressure (CPP). This hypothesis was originally widely accepted and was included in the US guidelines for the treatment of patients with severe traumatic brain lesions [2]. A contradictory view was presented from Lund, Sweden. According to Asgeirsson *et al.* reducing ICP was in these patients obtained by a pharmacologically induced *decrease* in MAP and CPP [3]. It seems highly unlikely both of these hypotheses are true. This review will examine the physiological and biochemical foundations of the two conflicting principles.

Except for decompressive craniectomy all treatments of increased ICP are directed towards decreasing the volume of one or more of the intracranial components:

$$V_{intracran} = V_{blood} + V_{brain} + V_{CSF} + V_{mass\ lesion}$$

Surgical treatments include evacuation of focal mass lesions ($V_{mass\ lesion}$) and, in selected cases, drainage of CSF (V_{CSF}). The importance of early and adequate surgical evacuation of focal mass lesions is well documented and will not be discussed further. The regulation of the remaining two volumes (V_{blood} and V_{brain}) is the target for non-surgical intensive care. The 'US – Rosner guidelines' for treatment of increased ICP [1,2] are exclusively directed towards decreasing V_{blood}, while the 'Lund concept' is mainly directed towards a decrease in V_{brain}.

The Vasonstrictor Cascade
The 'U.S. – Rosner concept' is based upon a hypothesis called the 'vasoconstrictor cascade' [1,4]. According to this hypothesis pressure autoregulation of cerebral blood flow is usually not abolished in patients with severe traumatic brain lesions but just shifted to the right (e.g. towards a higher MAP/CPP). A pharmacologically induced increase in MAP/CPP might then increase arterial blood pressure to within the new limits of autoregulation. When this level is reached

constriction of the precapillary resistance vessels will – according to this hypothesis – cause a decrease in intracranial blood volume (V_{blood}) and decrease ICP. The hypothesis has, however, several important weaknesses. It is well established that cerebral pressure autoregulation is often impaired in patients with head injuries [5] but it has never been convincingly demonstrated that the autoregulatory curve is shifted towards a higher MAP/CPP. More important, the blood volume within the precapillary resistance vessels is so minute that it is difficult to imagine that any volume change within this compartment would have any significant influence on ICP. Further, according to the Poiseuille-Hagen equation, flow is related to the radius of the vessel raised to the fourth power. This implies that very small changes in the diameter of the precapillary resistance vessels will have a very pronounced effect on blood flow. By definition pressure autoregulation means that blood flow remains unaffected when perfusion pressure changes and, accordingly, the decrease in the radius of the resistance vessels caused by the increase in CPP must be very small. Contrary to their assumptions regarding pressure autoregulation, all physiologically or pharmacologically induced constrictions of the precapillary resistance vessels that are known to decrease ICP (i.e. hypocapnia, hyperoxygenation, reduction of cerebral energy metabolism) do so by decreasing cerebral blood flow (CBF) and hence cerebral blood volume (CBV), the latter mainly within the venous compartment. Accordingly the 'vasoconstrictor cascade' does not appear to have a convincing physiological background. Further, the notion that an increase in CPP would cause a decrease in ICP is not supported by animal studies. In an experimental study of the injured feline brain, induced arterial hypertension invariably increased ICP [6].

Several authors have claimed that they have frequently observed a decrease in ICP during increases in CPP. However, in a prospective clinical study in head injured patients Oertel *et al.* [7] showed that hypocapnia as well as reduction of cerebral energy metabolism (both causing a decrease in CBF and CBV) were usually associated with a decrease in ICP while a pharmacologically induced increase in CPP almost invariable caused a further increase in ICP within 30 minutes. Thus, the physiological basis as well as the clinical support for the 'vasoconstrictor cascade' appears to be weak or absent.

Blood-brain barrier permeability and the 'Lund concept'
The 'Lund concept' is primarily based upon the physiological properties of the blood-brain barrier. Volume regulation of the brain is, like other organs, mainly determined by mechanisms controlling the water exchange across the capillaries. However, the brain differs

from all other organs in its highly sophisticated capillary membrane function, the blood-brain barrier. In addition to its other physiological functions the blood-brain barrier is the most important regulator of cerebral volume [8].

The flux of water across a membrane or microvascular bed (J_v) is described by the equation

$$J_v = L_p \times A \times [\Delta P - \Sigma \sigma_s \times \Delta \Pi_s]$$

where L_p is hydraulic conductivity, A is the surface area available for fluid exchange, ΔP is the transcapillary hydrostatic pressure difference, $\Delta \Pi_s$ the transcapillary osmotic pressure difference and σ_s the reflection coefficient of each solute (s) of the system. Transcapillary water transport is accordingly defined by the difference in hydrostatic pressure (ΔP), the osmotic pressure gradient ($\Delta \Pi_s$), the endothelial component which will determine which solutes are reflected and will contribute to the osmotic pressure gradient (σ_s), and the hydraulic conductance of the capillary wall ($L_p \times A$). The two major solutes of biological fluids (Na^+ and Cl^-) have a blood-brain barrier reflection coefficient of 1.0 (i.e. the blood-brain barrier is impermeable for these solutes). Water passing the blood-brain barrier in any direction will thus be virtually devoid of crystalloids and an opposing osmotic gradient, which counteracts further fluid movement, will immediately be created.

The magnitude of the hydraulic conductance ($L_p \times A$) describes the rate by which water is transferred across the capillary wall whenever there is a driving force ($\Delta P - \Sigma \sigma \times \Delta \Pi$). Accordingly, the only way of inducing transcapillary filtration or absorption is to influence the balance between the hydrostatic and osmotic forces across the capillary membrane. For two reasons, the magnitudes of the CPP and the intravascular colloid osmotic pressure are less important for brain volume regulation under normal conditions. Firstly, intracapillary hydrostatic pressure (and blood flow) is physiologically tightly autoregulated and variations in systemic blood pressure are generally not transmitted to cerebral capillaries. Secondly, transcapillary fluid exchange is effectively counteracted by the low permeability to crystalloids combined with the high osmotic pressure of approximately 5700 mmHg on both sides of the blood-brain barrier [8]. This contrasts to other capillary regions where the osmotic pressure force is mainly derived from the difference between plasma and interstitial colloid osmotic pressure approximately balancing the transcapillary hydrostatic pressure (20-25 mmHg). Under pathophysiological conditions, regulation of brain volume may be completely altered as pressure autoregulation is often impaired and the blood-brain barrier may have an increased permeability for crystalloids or even for large molecules. The regulation of brain volume will then depend on the balance between the transcapillary hydrostatic pressure and the transcapillary colloidal osmotic pressure (i.e. the Starling Equilibrium).

Pathophysiological aspects of disturbed brain volume regulation
There are no techniques are available for quantitative measurements of cerebral intracapillary hydrostatic pressure or the effects of increased hydrostatic pressure on water transport across the blood-brain barrier. However, some of these aspects have been studied in a model system using denervated cat skeletal muscle enclosed in a plethysmograph [9-12]. This model simulates the pathophysiological situation in a damaged brain since muscle capillaries are permeable for water and most solutes but much less permeable for proteins ($\sigma \sim 0.8\text{-}0.9$). Like in the injured brain pressure autoregulation of blood flow is impaired in this experimental model.

The clinical implications of these results may be summarised as follows: If the injured brain has an impaired pressure autoregulation and a blood-brain barrier with an increased permeability to crystalloids, then transcapillary fluid exchange will be highly dependent on variations in systemic arterial blood pressure. A decrease in arterial pressure will initially decrease CPP but, due to transcapillary fluid re-absorption, the slow decrease in tissue interstitial pressure (P_{tissue}) will restore CPP [11,12]. Further, if the blood brain barrier has an increased permeability to crystalloids, decreased P_{tissue} will cause a net transport of fluid from the capillaries into the interstitial space. All surgical treatments of increased ICP (evacuation of focal mass lesions, drainage of CSF, craniectomy) are associated with a decrease in P_{tissue}. This explains the pronounced brain swelling often observed after craniectomy.

The 'Lund concept'
The 'Lund concept' is based on these physiological principles and can be summarised in four paragraphs.

I. Reduction of stress response and cerebral energy metabolism
Stress response is reduced by liberal use of sedatives (benzodiazepines) and analgesics (opioids). A further reduction of the stress response and catecholamine release is obtained by a continuous infusion of low-dose thiopentone (0.5-3 mg/kg/hr), fentanyl (2-5 μg/kg/hr) and also with the β_1-antagonist metoprolol and the α_2-

agonist clonidine (see below). The dose of thiopentone is kept low to avoid cardiac inhibition, pulmonary complications and other side effects [13].

II. Reduction of capillary hydrostatic pressure

Mean arterial blood pressure is reduced to the physiological level for the age of the individual patient with an intravenous combination of metoprolol (0.2-0.3 mg/kg/24hr) and clonidine (0.4-0.8 µg/kg x 4-6 doses) [0,12,14,15]. The antihypertensive treatment is initiated after evacuation of focal mass lesions when the patients are normovolaemic as suggested by red cell and albumin / plasma transfusions to normal albumin and haemoglobin levels and central venous pressures. A CPP of 60-70 mmHg is usually considered optimal but, if necessary to control ICP, a transient decrease in CPP to 50 mmHg for adults and 40 mmHg for children is acceptable. Thiopentone also has a precapillary vasoconstrictor effect, which will contribute to lowering the intracapillary hydrostatic pressure.

III. Maintenance of colloid osmotic pressure and control of fluid balance

Red cell transfusions and albumin are given to achieve normal values (12.5-14.0 g/dl and ~ 40 g/l, respectively) to ensure normovolemia and to optimise oxygen supply. The albumin / plasma / blood transfusions also help maintaining a normal colloid osmotic pressure favouring transcapillary absorption. A balanced or moderately negative fluid balance is a part of the treatment protocol and is achieved by diuretics (furosemide) and albumin infusion. All patients are given a low calorie enteral nutrition (max energy supply 15-20 kcal/kg/day).

IV. Reduction of cerebral blood volume

The principles discussed above constitute the corner-stone of the Lund concept but the protocol also includes measures to decrease CBV. The patients are always kept sedated with controlled ventilation to a normal $PaCO_2$; hyperventilation is used only for short-term decrease in ICP. Further, cerebral blood volume may also be reduced both on the arterial side with low-dose thiopentone [12,16] and on the venous side with dihydroergotamine [12,17-19]. Dihydroergotamine is only given when other treatments (above) are insufficient and always at the lowest dose necessary to reduce intracranial pressure. In practice, dihydroergotamine is rarely used. When given it is never administered for more than five days in order to minimize the risks of compromising peripheral circulation, in particular in patients with fractures of the extremities or renal insufficiency. The maximum doses of dihydroergotamine used are: 0.8 µg/kg/hr on day one, 0.6

µg/kg/hr on day two, 0.4 µg/kg/hr on day three, 0.2 µg/kg/hr on day four, and 0.1 µg/kg/hr on day five.

Intracerebral microdialysis
The 'Lund concept' does risk promoting secondary brain damage. Reducing CPP in patients with increased ICP might jeopardize cerebral energy metabolism in particular in the penumbra zones surrounding focal mass lesions. To avoid secondary adverse events, intracerebral microdialysis may help. Variables reflecting cerebral energy metabolism and cell membrane degradation can be analyzed and displayed at the bedside.

Microdialysis was introduced more than 25 years ago for monitoring the animal brain [20,21] and has become a standard technique in neuroscience with well over 11000 publications. In 1995, CMA Microdialysis (Stockholm, Sweden) introduced microdialysis instruments for clinical use (catheters for peripheral and brain tissue, a microdialysis pump, and a bedside chemical analyzer). This new clinical instrument was initially used to monitor patients treated according to the 'Lund concept' [22,23]. The first microdialysis catheter designed for human brain consisted of a 60 mm long shaft and a 10 mm long dialysis membrane (polyamide; 20000 molecular weight cutoff) with an outer diameter of 0.62 mm. The microdialysis catheters are perfused with a Ringer solution at 0.3 µl/min from a micro infusion pump. The microdialysis samples are collected in capped micro vials to prevent evaporation and analyzed at the bedside using ordinary enzymatic methods. The chemical variables of particular interest during intensive care are those related to glycolysis (glucose, pyruvate, lactate), degradation of the glycerophopholipids of cell membranes (glycerol), and excessive levels of excitatory transmitters (glutamate). A simplified diagram of intermediary metabolism as well as the reference levels in normal human brain is shown in Figure 1.

The measured levels of the chemical substances correspond to their absolute interstitial concentrations only if a complete equilibration has occurred through the dialysis membrane. The degree of equilibration for a permeable substance (relative recovery) is mainly dependent on the perfusion rate, the length of the dialysis membrane and the diffusion of the substance in the tissue. When the microdialysis technique is used clinically the estimated recoveries of the monitored variables (glucose, pyruvate, lactate, glycerol, glutmate) are about 70% of their true interstitial levels [24]. However, recovery may vary in different pathophysiological situations due to changed conditions for diffusion in the tissue. This variability is of relevance when

CRITICAL CARE FOCUS 14: UPDATES

Figure 1. Simplified diagram of cerebral intermediary metabolism of the glycolytic chain and its relation to the formation of glycerol and glycerophospholipids and to the citric acid cycle. F-1,6-DP: Fructose-1,6-diposphate; DHAP: Dihydroxyacetone-phosphate; GA-3P: Glyceraldehyde-3-phosphate; G-3-P: Glycerol-3-phosphate; FFA: Free fatty acids; α-KG: α-ketoglutarate. Underlined metabolites are measured bedside with enzymatic techniques. References levels of the various metabolites for normal human brain obtained from Ref 26.

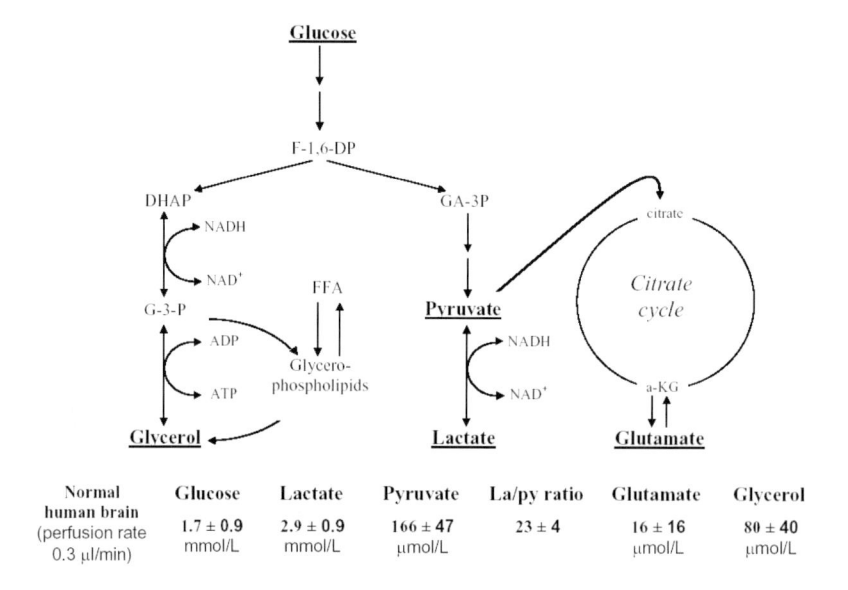

Normal human brain (perfusion rate 0.3 μl/min)	Glucose	Lactate	Pyruvate	La/py ratio	Glutamate	Glycerol
	1.7 ± 0.9 mmol/L	2.9 ± 0.9 mmol/L	166 ± 47 μmol/L	23 ± 4	16 ± 16 μmol/L	80 ± 40 μmol/L

performing studies of absolute concentration levels (e.g. pharmacokinetic studies) [25]. However, during intensive care the changes caused by perturbation of energy metabolism are so profound that minor changes in relative recovery are of no importance. Figure 1 gives the reference levels for normal human brain for the variables monitored during routine neurointensive care [26]. The level of glycerol and the lactate:pyruvate ratio are usually of particular clinical interest. A marked increase in intracerebral glycerol indicates degradation of the glycerophospholipids of the cell membranes [27-29]. The lactate:pyruvate ratio gives the lactate dehydrogenase equilibrium, which reflects the cytoplasmatic redox state [30]:

$$\frac{[NADH] \times [H^+]}{[NAD^+]} = \frac{[Lactate]}{[Pyruvate]} \times K_{LDH}$$

The microdialysis technique gives biochemical information only from a small volume surrounding the catheter. This is often an advantage during neurointensive care since most adverse events initially affect

THE LUND APPROACH

only the penumbra zones surrounding focal lesions [31,32]. Consequently it is necessary to insert the microdialysis catheters into these areas of interest and to document (by CT scanning) that the catheters have been correctly positioned. Figure 2 illustrates that one microdialysis catheter (M.D. 1) may be positioned in the 'penumbra zone' surrounding an evacuated focal brain contusion while the second catheter (M.D. 2) may be placed in the contralateral (better) hemisphere.

Figure 2. Median level (central square) for the lactate/pyruvate (la/py) ratio (n: 7,704; logarithmic scale) in the 'better' and 'worse' positions in relation to four ranges of CPP. The boxes (filled – better; open – worse) represent the lower and the upper quartile and the whiskers represent range. The CT-scans show the positioning of the microdialysis catheters in the 'worse' (M.D. 1) and 'better' (M.D. 2) parts of the brain as well as the ventricular catheter (V.C.). Data from Ref 33.

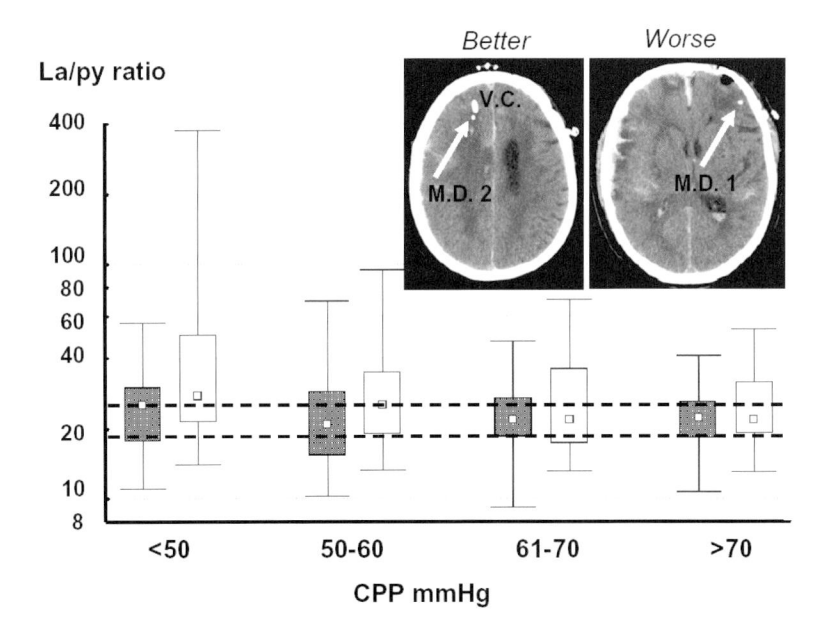

Intracerebral microdialysis is used routinely to monitor patients during the reduction in MAP/CPP induced according to the 'Lund concept'. The cytoplasmatic red-ox state (lactate:pyruvate ratio) will increase instantaneously and recover rapidly during a period of transient ischemia. Figure 2 shows median levels for the lactate/pyruvate ratio (n = 7704) in the 'better' and 'worse' positions in relation to four ranges of CPP in as series of severely head-injured patients [33]. The median levels are given by the central squares, the boxes (filled –

101

better; open – worse) represent the lower and the upper quartile, and the whiskers represent range. The normal human intracerebral lactate:pyruvate ratio (mean 23 ± standard deviation 4) is indicated by the interrupted lines [26]. No statistically significant difference in lactate:pyruvate ratio was obtained when comparing the 'worse' and 'better' positions at CPP>70 mmHg. The lactate:pyruvate ratio was higher (p=0.04) in the 'worse' than in the 'better' position at CPP <50 mmHg. When comparing CPP <50 mmHg to CPP >70 mmHg and CPP <50 mmHg to CPP >50 mmHg the lactate:pyruvate ratio was higher at the low CPP in the worse position (p=0.04 and p=0.01, respectively). No difference in lactate:pyruvate ratio was obtained in the 'better' position when comparing CPP <50 mmHg to CPP >50 mmHg.

Figure 3. Reduction of mean arterial blood pressure (MAP; mean ± Standard Error of the Meam (SEM)) and cerebral perfusion pressure (CPP; mean ± SEM) during the first 72 hours after start of treatment according to the 'Lund concept'. Data from Ref 23.

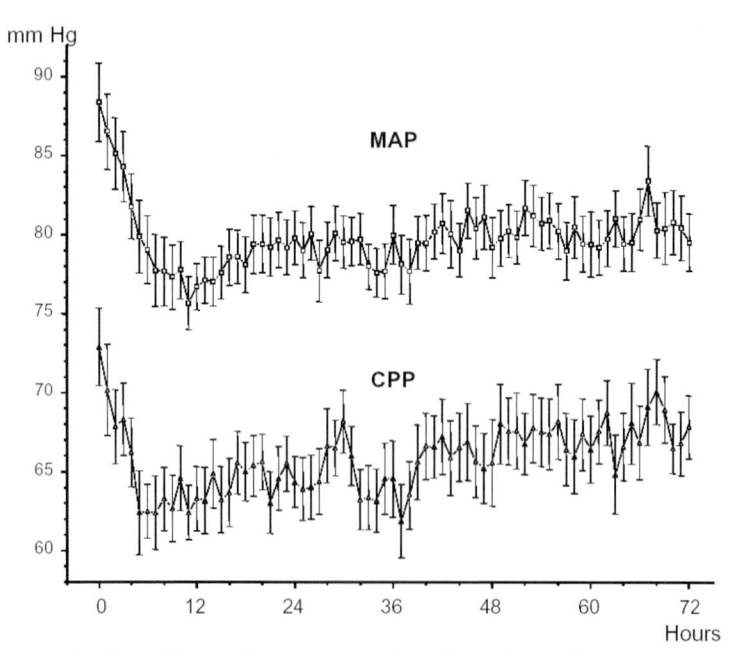

In conclusion this study supports the view that, if necessary for the treatment of increased ICP, CPP might be reduced to 50 mmHg provided the physiological and pharmacological principles of the 'Lund concept' are recognized. However, it must be recognized that variations between patients might be considerable. In the individual patient preservation of normal cerebral energy metabolism within areas at risk could be protected by intracerebral microdialysis and adjustment of the desired level of CPP.

Biochemical evaluation of tissue outcome
The efficacy of therapy given during neuro intensive care is conventionally judged from evaluation of clinical outcome. The microdialysis technique offers an additional possibility; the biochemical restitution of energy metabolism and intermediary metabolism may be used as an indicator of 'tissue outcome'. It is then of particular interest to monitor biochemical restitution in the vulnerable penumbra zones [31,32].

Figures 3 and 4 summarise the physiological and biochemical information in a series of patients treated according to the 'Lund concept' [23]. Figure 3 shows changes in MAP and CPP during the first 72 hours after start of treatment and Figure 4 gives the simultaneously obtained intracerebral glycerol levels in the 'worse' and 'better' parts of the brain. Due to the pharmacologically induced reduction in MAP the CPP initially decreased from 73 to 62 mmHg (Figure 3). The capillary re-absorption of interstitial fluid caused a gradual decrease in ICP and a slow increase in CPP back to 65-70 mmHg. The pharmacologically induced decrease in CPP was associated with a simultaneous decrease in interstitial glycerol in the 'worse' from a very high level (>300 µmol/L) at the start of treatment to normal level within 72 hours (Figure 4). These data supports the view that the vulnerable penumbra zone tolerates a controlled decrease in CPP provided it is achieved according to the physiological principles discussed above.

The 'Lund concept' – clinical results
Ideally all clinical therapies should be based on randomised controlled studies. However, there are virtually no such studies to support any specific treatment for increased ICP [34-37]. There is only one published randomised clinical trial showing the consequences of targeting different levels of CPP in patients with severe brain trauma. This study failed to show a long-term benefit of increasing CPP above 70 mmHg [38]. The US guidelines recommendations to keep CPP very high are probably slowly changing and in a recent review on the management of cerebral perfusion pressure after head trauma it was concluded that it seemed likely that a CPP of 60 mmHg provided adequate perfusion for most patients with severe traumatic brain injuries [39]. The clinical outcome in patients treated for severe traumatic brain injury according to the 'Lund-concept' has been reported from four Swedish neurosurgical centres [40-43]. All four studies have shown a remarkably low mortality. In the original study,

Figure 4. Glycerol levels (mean ± SEM) obtained bedside from microdialysis catheters in the penumbra zone surrounding evacuated focal brain lesions (Glycerol worse) as well as from the contralateral 'better' hemisphere (Glycerol better). The interrupted lines indicate the range (mean ± S.D.) in normal human brain during wakefulness [26]. The simultaneous physiological data are shown in figure 3. The intentional decrease in CPP was associated with a normalization of all studied biochemical variables. Data from Ref 23.

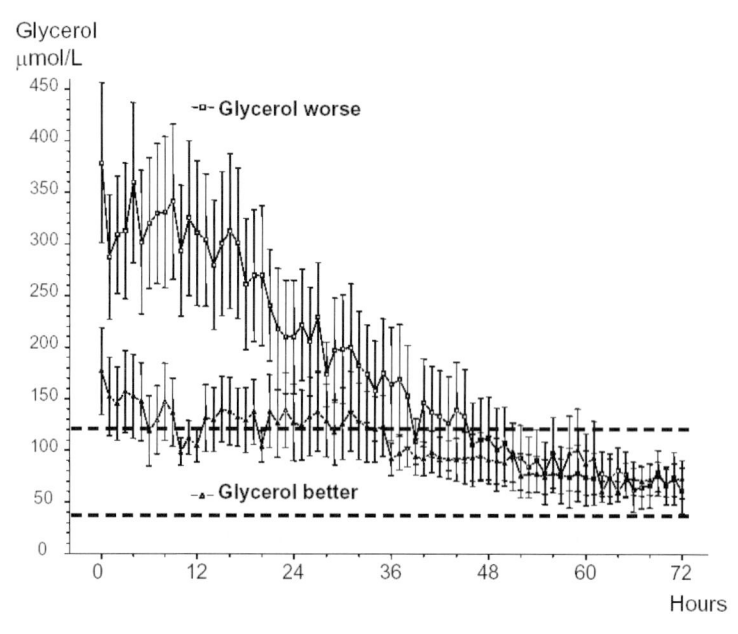

which included a selected group of patients with very severe traumatic brain lesion and ICP above 25 mmHg in spite of conventional treatment, the decrease in mortality was from 47% to 8% [40]. The significant decrease in mortality was associated with significant increases in the groups of 'good recovery' and 'moderate disability' but did not increase the number of patients in the groups of 'severe disability' or 'vegetative state'.

Conclusion

The 'Lund concept' is mainly directed towards increasing the re-absorption of cerebral interstitial water by 1) reduction of stress response and cerebral energy metabolism, 2) reduction of capillary hydrostatic pressure, 3) maintenance of colloid osmotic pressure and control of fluid balance. The efficacy of the treatment protocol has been evaluated in experimental and clinical studies regarding the physiological and biochemical (utilizing intracerebral microdialysis) effects. The clinical experiences have been favourable.

References

1. Rosner MJ, Rosner SD, Johnson AH. Cerebral perfusion pressure: Management protocol and clinical results. Journal of Neurosurgery 1995; 83: 949-962.
2. Asgeirsson B, Grände PO, Nordström CH. A new therapy of post-trauma brain oedema based on haemodynamic principles for brain volume regulation. Intensive Care Medicine 1994; 20: 260-267.
3. Bullock R, Chesnut RM, Clifton G, *et al*. Guidelines for the management of severe head injury. European Journal of Emergency Medicine 1996; 3: 109-127.
4. Rosner MJ, Becker DP. Origin and evolution of plateau waves. Experimental observations and a theoretical model. Journal of Neurosurgery 1984; 60: 312-324.
5. Cold GE, Jensen FT. Cerebral autoregulation in unconscious patients with brain injury. Acta Anaesthesiologica Scandinavica 1978; 22: 270-280.
6. Kongstad L, Grände PO. Arterial hypertension increases intracranial pressure in cat after opening of the blood-brain barrier. Journal of Trauma 2001; 51: 490-496.
7. Oertel M, Kelly DF, Lee JH, *et al*. Efficacy of hyperventilation, blood pressure elevation, and metabolic suppression therapy in controlling intracranial pressure after head injury. Journal of Neurosurgery 2002; 97: 1045-1053.
8. Fenstermacher JD. Volume regulation of the central nervous system. In *Edema*, ed. Staub NC, Taylor AE. New York: Raven Press, 1984, pp 383-404.
9. Asgeirsson B, Grände PO. Effects of arterial and venous pressure alterations on transcapillary fluid exchange during raised tissue pressure. Intensive Care Medicine 1994; 20: 567-572.
10. Grände PO, Asgeirsson B, Nordström CH. Physiological principles for volume regulation of a tissue enclosed in a rigid shell with application to the injured brain. Journal of Trauma 1997; 42: S23-S31.
11. Kongstad L, Grände PO. The role of arterial and venous pressure for volume regulation of an organ enclosed in a rigid compartment with application to the injured brain. Acta Anaesthesiologica Scandinavica 1999; 43: 501-508.
12. Grände PO, Asgeirsson B, Nordström CH. Volume targeted therapy of increased intracranial pressure: the Lund concept unifies surgical and non-surgical treatments. Acta Anaesthesiologica Scandinavica 2002; 46: 929-941.
13. Schalén W, Messeter K, Nordström CH. Complications and side effects during thiopentone therapy in patients with severe head injuries. Acta Anaesthesiologica Scandinavica 1992; 36: 369-377.

14. Asgeirsson B, Grände PO, Nordström CH. A new therapy of post-trauma brain oedema based on haemodynamic principles for brain volume regulation. Intensive Care Medicine 1994; 20: 260-267.
15. Asgeirsson B, Grände PO, Nordström CH, et al. Effects of hypotensive treatment with α_2-agonist and β_1-antagonist on cerebral hemodynamics in severe head injury. Acta Anaesthesiologica Scandinavica 1995; 39: 347-351.
16. Nordström CH, Messeter K, Sundbärg G, et al. Cerebral blood flow, vasoreactivity, and oxygen consumption during barbiturate therapy in severe traumatic brain lesions. Journal of Neurosurgery 1988; 68: 424-431.
17. Asgeirsson B, Grände PO, Nordström CH, et al. Cerebral hemodynamic effects of dihydroergotamine in patients with intracranial hypertension after severe head injury. Acta Anaesthesiologica Scandinavica 1995; 39: 922-930.
18. Nilsson F, Messeter K, Grände PO, et al. Effects of dihydroergotamine on cerebral circulation during experimental intracranial hypertension. Acta Anaesthesiologica Scandinavica 1995; 39: 916-921.
19. Nilsson F, Nilsson T, Edvinsson L, et al. Effects of dihydroergotamine and sumatriptan on isolated human cerebral and peripheral arteries and veins. Acta Anaesthesiologica Scandinavica 1997; 41:1257-1262.
20. Ungerstedt U, Pycock CH. Functional correlates of dopamine neurotransmission. Bulletin der Schweiz Akademie der Medizinischen Wissenschaften 1974; 30: 44-55.
21. Ungerstedt U. Microdialysis – principles and application for studies in animal and man. Journal of Internal Medicine 1991; 230: 365-373.
22. Ståhl N, Mellergård P, Hallström Å, et al. Intracerebral microdialysis and bedside biochemical analysis in patients with fatal traumatic brain lesions. Acta Anaesthesiologica Scandinavica 2001; 45: 977-985.
23. Ståhl N, Ungerstedt U, Nordström CH. Brain energy metabolism during controlled reduction of cerebral perfusion pressure in severe head injuries. Intensive Care Medicine 2001; 27: 1215-1223.
24. Hutchinson PJ, O'Connell MT, al-Rawi PG, et al. Clinical cerebral microdialysis - determining the true extracellular concentration. Acta Neurochirurgica Supplement 2002; 81: 359-362.
25. Ederoth P, Tunblad K, Bouw R, et al. Blood-brain barrier transport of morphine in patients with severe brain trauma. British Journal fo Clinical Pharmacology 2004; 57: 427-435.
26. Reinstrup P, Ståhl N, Hallström Å, et al. Intracerebral microdialysis in clinical practice. Normal values and variations

during anaesthesia and neurosurgical operations. Neurosurgery 2000; 47: 701-710.
27. Nordström C-H, Ungerstedt U. Intracerebral microdialysis with bedside analysis of lactate, glucose, glycerol and urea. In *Brain protection in severe head injury*, ed. Diemath HE. München: W Zuckswerdt Verlag, 1996, pp 117-119.
28. Ungerstedt U, Bäckström T, Hallström Å, *et al*. Microdialysis in normal and injured human brain. In *Physiology, stress, and malnutrition*, ed. Kinney JM, Tucker H. Philadelphia: Lippincott - Raven Publishers, 1997, pp 361-374.
29. Hillered L, Valtysson J, Enblad P, *et al*. Interstitial glycerol as a marker for membrane phospholipid degradation in the acutely injured human brain. Journal of Neurology, Neurosurgery, and Psychiatry 1998; 64: 486-491.
30. Siesjö BK. *Brain Energy Metabolism*. Chichester: John Wiley & Sons, 1978.
31. Ståhl N, Schalén W, Ungerstedt U, *et al*. Bedside biochemical monitoring of the penumbra zone surrounding an evacuated acute subdural haematoma. Acta Neurologica Scandinavica 2003; 108: 211-215.
32. Engström M, Polito A, Reinstrup P, *et al*. Intracerebral microdialysis in clinical routine – the importance of catheter location. Journal of Neurosurgery 2005; 102: 460-469.
33. Nordström CH, Reinstrup P, Xu W, *et al*. Assessment of the lower limit for cerebral perfusion pressure in severe head injuries by bedside monitoring of regional energy metabolism. Anesthesiology 2003; 98: 809-814.
34. Roberts I, Schierhout G. Hyperventilation therapy for acute traumatic brain injury. *Cochrane Database of Systematic Reviews* 1997, Issue 4. Art. No.: CD000566. DOI: 10.1002/14651858.CD000566.
35. Roberts I. Barbiturates for acute traumatic brain injury. *Cochrane Database of Systematic Reviews* 1997, Issue 3. Art. No.: CD000033. DOI: 10.1002/14651858.CD000033.
36. Wakai A, Roberts I, Schierhout G. Mannitol for acute traumatic brain injury. *Cochrane Database of Systematic Reviews* 1998, Issue 1. Art. No.: CD001049. DOI: 10.1002/14651858.CD001049.pub4.
37. Alderson P, Roberts I. Corticosteroids for acute traumatic brain injury. *Cochrane Database of Systematic Reviews* 1997, Issue 3. Art. No.: CD000196. DOI: 10.1002/14651858.CD000196.pub2.
38. Robertson CS, Valadka AB, Hannay J, *et al*. Prevention of secondary ischemic insults after severe head injury. Critical Care Medicine 1999; 27: 2086-2095.

39. Robertson CS. Management of cerebral perfusion pressure after traumatic brain injury. Anesthesiology 2001; 95: 1513-1517.
40. Eker C, Asgeirsson B, Grände PO, *et al*. Improved outcome after severe head injury with a new therapy based on principles for brain volume regulation and improved microcirculation. Critical Care Medicine 1998; 26: 1881-1886.
41. Naredi S, Edén E, Zäll S, *et al*. A standardized neurosurgical/neurointensive therapy directed toward vasogenic edema after severe traumatic brain injury: clinical results. Intensive Care Medicine 1998; 24: 446-451.
42. Naredi S, Olivecrona M, Lindgren A, *et al*. An outcome study of severe traumatic head injury using the 'Lund therapy' with low-dose prostacyclin. Acta Anaesthesiologica Scandinavica 2001; 45: 401-405.
43. Elf K, Nilsson P, Enblad P. Outcome after traumatic brain injury improved by an organized secondary insult program and standardized neurointensive care. Critical Care Medicine 2002; 30: 2129-2134.

8: Temperature Reduction after Acute Brain injury

DR MANOJ SAXENA, PROF PETER ANDREWS, MS BRIDGET HARRIS and DR OLAV THULESIUS

Introduction

Acute brain injury is a frequent cause of disability and death worldwide and commonly occurs in perinatal asphyxia, traumatic brain injury, stroke and out of hospital cardiac arrest. It affects patients of all ages. Interruption of cerebral oxygen and nutrient delivery by cardiorespiratory insufficiency or vascular occlusion may precipitate cerebral ischaemia. The initial pathology may not induce immediate cell death, but can trigger a complex biochemical cascade leading to delayed neuronal loss increasing the risk of death or disability (Figure 1). This chapter reviews the current evidence for temperature reduction after neuronal injury.

Figure 1. Inflammatory pathological events after acute brain injury. Injury activates microglia cells and astrocytes to release cytokines & eventually lead to tangle and plaque formation with neuro-degeneration, memory deficits and Alzheimer's disease.

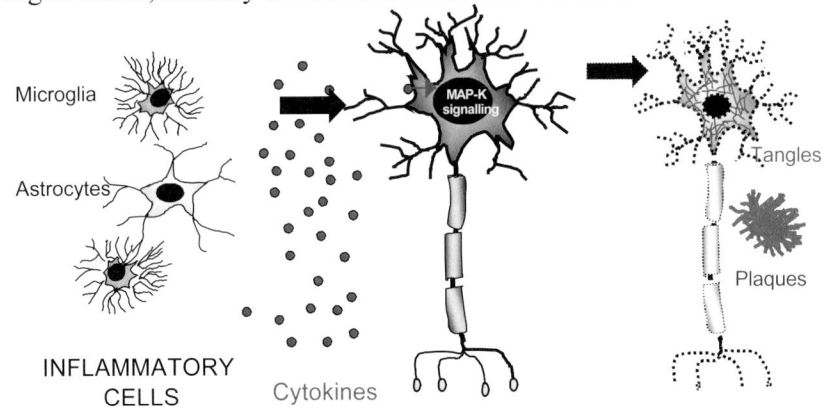

Background

Preclinical studies have demonstrated that temperature reduction before, during and after experimental neurological injury improves outcomes. A recent systematic review of hypothermia in animal models of acute ischaemic stroke suggested that infarct volume could be reduced by 44% (95% confidence interval (CI) 40% - 47%) with cooling to 31 °C. Temperature reduction to only 35 °C also appeared to substantially reduce infarct volume (30%, 95% CI 21 - 39%), suggesting that smaller temperature reductions may still have clinically worthwhile effects (personal communication Dr Malcolm McLeod, Consultant Neurologist, Stirling Royal Infirmary, UK) with less challenging temperature reduction.

We believe that there are two distinct clinical hypotheses that require separate evaluation. Firstly, can temperature reduction to 32-34 °C (mild systemic hypothermia) improve clinical outcomes if applied in the first minutes to hours after neuronal injury? There is evidence to support this hypothesis in adults following cardiac arrest and in neonates following perinatal hypoxia. Secondly, in the days immediately after neuronal injury can preventing pyrexia reduce neuronal injury and improve clinical outcomes? Interventions preventing pyrexia in the first days after neuronal injury may have wider application because it is easier to administer. Hence, even a small absolute benefit achieved by preventing pyrexia would potentially avoid many deaths and disabilities worldwide. Similarly, because some of these strategies are already widely used in an *ad hoc* manner after neuronal injuries, demonstrating lack of any benefit would protect patients from an unnecessary intervention and its associated side-effects and costs.

Early temperature reduction to 32-34 °C (mild systemic hypothermia) and clinical outcomes.

There are many techniques for delivering systemic hypothermia including air or water-circulating surface cooling blankets, endovascular cooling systems with catheter placement in the inferior vena cava [1] and ice-cold intravenous fluids [2, 3]. The main advantage of systemic hypothermia is that target core temperatures can be achieved rapidly. However, systemic hypothermia has side-effects and also requires staff expertise and additional equipment. It is therefore both complex and expensive.

The effects of systemic hypothermia on platelet function and coagulation may be a concern in the early phase of traumatic brain injury, intracerebral or subarachnoid haemorrhage. Maintaining systemic hypothermia during transfers and other investigations can be challenging. To help achieve core temperatures between 32-34 °C, it may be necessary to anaesthetise the patient on intensive care. This increases the complexity and the cost of the intervention further so limiting the patient population to which this strategy may be applied.

Additional complications of systemic cooling include immunosuppression, infection, cold induced diuresis, electrolyte imbalances and shivering [4]. A hyperadrenergic state is present after

MANAGEMENT OF HEAD INJURY

traumatic brain injury and hypothermia may paradoxically aggravate this condition.

Even so systemic hypothermia in the early phase after neuronal injury warrants further investigation. However trials in cardiac arrest [5-7] and perinatal asphyxia [8, 9] may be difficult to replicate in patients with traumatic brain injury, stroke and subarachnoid haemorrhage. After cardiac arrest and perinatal asphyxia, patients reach health care services rapidly and do not pose a diagnostic or therapeutic dilemma. In these situations, mild hypothermia may be implemented shortly after neuronal injury as the therapeutic benefit of systemic hypothermia decreases with increasing time from neuronal injury. In other conditions, there may be a longer time from injury to cooling because of diagnostic uncertainty.

There have been several recent systematic reviews of traumatic brain injury [10-13]. The major issues in these reviews include heterogeneity of inclusion criteria, time to target temperature, degree and duration of hypothermia, re-warming methods and management of the control groups. With the exception of McIntyre's review in 2003 which concluded that hypothermia may reduce the risk of mortality after traumatic brain injury [13], other reviews have suggested that there is little evidence for the use of therapeutic hypothermia at present.

A recent Cochrane review of cooling therapies after acute stroke (ischaemic and intracerebral haemorrhage, but not including subarachnoid haemorrhage) did not identify any completed randomised controlled studies [14]. We have recently carried out a systematic review of cooling therapies after subarachnoid haemorrhage (in press) and this also failed to identify any randomised controlled trials.

Therefore in summary, there are no randomised controlled clinical trials that support the use of mild systemic hypothermia after stroke, subarachnoid haemorrhage or traumatic brain injury. It may be a significant challenge to replicate the promising data demonstrated following cardiac arrest and perinatal asphyxia in other patient populations.

In the days immediately after neuronal injury can preventing pyrexia reduce neuronal injury and improve clinical outcomes.
Cooling the brain parenchyma is logical since brain rather than trunk temperature is important in cerebral protection [15, 16]. In a foetal model of brain asphyxia, direct brain cooling showed a reduction in

neuronal loss throughout deep brain structures. A cooling cap placed on the cranium of a piglet [15] achieved a significant temperature reduction in both superficial and deep structures of the brain [17, 18]. Therefore it was concluded that direct brain cooling might be effective for cerebral resuscitation in paediatric practice. Thulesius *et al* have designed a neck collar perfused with cooled glycol (-1 to -4 ^{0}C) to induce cooling and vasodilatation of the carotid artery [19-21]. Calculations based on a theoretical model have shown that neck cooling of arterial blood can achieve 1.1 ^{0}C reduction in brain temperature [22]. In human thermoregulatory research, there is also some experimental data to support direct brain cooling [22-24]. Liu *et al* suggests that the combination of general hypothermia and direct brain cooling may offer some advantages.

In Edinburgh two randomised controlled direct brain cooling trials have been conducted in brain injured intubated patients. In the first trial, air continually flowed through both nostrils at equivalent to normal minute ventilation. This did not produce any direct brain cooling as measured by a Camino pressure/ temperature monitor placed in the frontal cortex. [25]. However, a subsequent trial [26] where nasal air flow and head fanning were performed alone and in combination did show evidence of direct brain cooling with a mean brain temperature fall of 0.41 ^{0}C after 30 minutes.

Therefore, direct brain cooling may be achieved by conductive cooling of the neck and/or convective cooling using simple fans and other devices that optimise airflow and heat loss from the scalp [27, 28]. These non-invasive techniques require further evaluation in terms of both feasibility and efficacy. They could test the hypothesis that preventing pyrexia in the first few days after neuronal injury may beneficially modulate patient outcome and subsequently have potentially wide application [29, 30] (in conjunction with supportive care and medication, see below).

In an observational study of patients with acute stroke, increased body temperature was associated with large lesion volumes, high case fatality, and poor functional outcome. Reith and colleagues demonstrated in a prospective observational study that a 1 ^{0}C increase in body temperature after stroke increases the odds of a poor outcome by a factor of 2.2 [31, 32]. These data suggested that interventions that reduce temperatures of this magnitude after stroke warrant further evaluation (Table 1).

Table 1. Methods of direct brain cooling. For more details, see Harris BA Andrews PJD. Direct Brain Cooling In: *Hypothermia in Neurocritical Care*. Eds, Mayer SA & Sessler DI. Marcel Dekker: New York. 2004, Chapter 11.

Non-invasive methods
- heat loss from the upper airways – nasal gas flow and lavage
- heat loss through the skull – external forced convection (fanning, cooling hoods) and conduction (cooling caps)

Invasive methods
- antegrade cerebral perfusion - unilateral femoral / carotid bypass via a heat exchanger
- intracarotid flush - a cold solution, usually at 0 °C but 2, 4 or 8 °C is pumped into one common carotid artery for five or six minutes at a rate of 10 ml/kg/min
- open and semi-closed irrigation - cooling by irrigation of the brain surface
- contact cooling of specific areas of the brain - circulating cold fluid through open-ended Teflon capsules placed in burr holes or through tubing laid on the brain surface and use of sacs filled with gas cooled liquid placed directly on the brain surface.

Pharmacology

Anti-pyretic drugs include paracetamol (acetaminophen), non-steroidal anti-inflammatory drugs and selective cyclo-oxygenase inhibitors. However, concerns about the anti-platelet effect of the latter drug types may limit their use in brain injury. Dippel *et al* have argued that paracetamol induced tympanic temperature falls of 0.27 °C may reduce the relative risk of poor outcome after acute ischaemic stroke by 10-20% [33, 34]. The risk of a poor outcome has also been found to rise by a factor of 2.2 for each degree centigrade increase in body temperature (95% CI 1.4 - 3.5) after acute ischaemic stroke [35, 36]. Two randomised double blind clinical trials in patients with acute ischaemic stroke have recently shown that treatment with a daily dose of 6 g paracetamol results in a small but rapid and potentially worthwhile reduction of 0.3 °C (95% CI: 0.1-0.5 °C) in body temperature. There is a large multi-centre randomized controlled clinical trial underway exploring whether 1 g of paracetamol given every 4 hours over 3 days to patients with acute ischaemic stroke improves patient outcome (www.strokecenter.org/trials & www.pais-study.org/).

Drug therapy and the techniques of direct brain cooling have independent mechanisms of action and hence may have additive effects. Together they may provide temperature reduction of an order of magnitude that may be clinically important. This requires formal evaluation.

Conclusion

Today several different methods of temperature reduction are available for the treatment of brain injured patients. Therapeutic hypothermia in the immediate hours after neuronal injury has been found to be neuroprotective in animal models, as well as in clinical studies after cardiac arrest and perinatal asphyxia. Direct brain cooling and drug therapy may be better suited to answering whether preventing pyrexia in the first days after neuronal injury can improve patient outcomes. Both interventions warrant further investigation.

References

1. Furuse M, Ohta T, Ikenaga T, *et al.* Effects of intravascular perfusion of cooled crystalloid solution on cold-induced brain injury using an extracorporeal cooling-filtration system. Acta Neurochirurgica 2003; 145: 983-992.
2. Polderman KH, Rijnsburger ER, Peerdeman SM, Girbes ARJ. Induction of hypothermia in patients with various types of neurologic injury with use of large volumes of ice-cold intravenous fluid. Critical Care Medicine 2005; 33: 2744-2751.
3. Bernard SA, Buist M. Induced hypothermia in critical care medicine: A review. Critical Care Medicine 2003; 31: 2041-2051.
4. Polderman KH, Girbes AR. Severe electrolyte disorders following cardiac surgery: a prospective controlled observational study. Critical Care 2004; 8: R459-R466.
5. Bernard SA, Gray TW, Buist MD, *et al.* Treatment of comatose survivors of out-of-hospital cardiac arrest with induced hypothermia. New England Journal of Medicine 2002; 346: 557-563.
6. Holzer M, Sterz F and Hypothermia After Cardiac Arrest Study Group. Therapeutic hypothermia after cardiopulmonary resuscitation. Expert Review of Cardiovascular Therapy 2003; 1: 317-325.
7. Hypothermia After Cardiac Arrest Study Group. Mild therapeutic hypothermia to improve the neurologic outcome after cardiac arrest. New England Journal of Medicine 2002; 346: 549-556.
8. Gunn AJ, Thoresen M. Hypothermic neuroprotection. NeuroRx 2006; 3: 154-169.
9. Lin ZL, Yu HM, Lin J, Chen SQ, Liang ZQ, Zhang ZY. Mild hypothermia via selective head cooling as neuroprotective therapy in term neonates with perinatal asphyxia: An experience from a

single neonatal intensive care unit. Journal of Perinatology 2006; 26: 180-184.
10. Harris OA, Colford JM Jr, Good MC, Matz PG. The role of hypothermia in the management of severe brain injury: a meta-analysis. Archives of Neurology 2002; 59: 1077-1083.
11. Henderson WR, Dhingra VK, Chittock DR, Fenwick JC, Ronco JJ. Hypothermia in the management of traumatic brain injury. A systematic review and meta-analysis. Intensive Care Medicine 2003; 29: 1637-1644.
12. Alderson P, Gadkary C, Signorini DF. Therapeutic hypothermia for head injury. Cochrane Database of Systematic Reviews, 2004. http://www.cochrane.org/reviews/en/ab001048.html
13. McIntyre LA, Fergusson DA, Hebert PC, Moher D, Hutchison JS. Prolonged therapeutic hypothermia after traumatic brain injury in adults: A systematic review. Journal of the American Medical Association 2003; 289: 2992-2999.
14. Correia M, Silva M, Veloso M. Cooling therapy for acute stroke. Cochrane Database of Systematic Reviews, 2006. Issue 3. http://www.update-software.com/abstracts/AB001247.htm
15. Gelman B, Schleien CL, Lohe A, Kuluz JW. Selective brain cooling in infant piglets after cardiac arrest and resuscitation. Critical Care Medicine 24: 1009-1017.
16. Hagioka S, Takeda Y, Takata K, Morita K. Nasopharyngeal cooling selectively and rapidly decreases brain temperature and attenuates neuronal damage, even if initiated at the onset of cardiopulmonary resuscitation in rats. Critical Care Medicine 2003; 31: 2502-2508.
17. Laptook AR, Shalak L, Corbett RJ. Differences in brain temperature and cerebral blood flow during selective head versus whole-body cooling. Pediatrics 2001; 108: 1103-1110.
18. Laptook AR, Corbett RJ. The effects of temperature on hypoxic-ischemic brain injury. Clinics in Perinatology 2002; 29: 623-649.
19. Mustafa S, Thulesius O. Cooling-induced carotid artery dilatation: An experimental study in isolated vessels. Stroke 2002; 33: 256-260.
20. Mustafa S, Thulesius O, Ismael HN. Hyperthermia-induced vasoconstriction of the carotid artery, a possible causative factor of heatstroke. Journal of Applied Physiology 2004; 96: 1875-1878.
21. Mustafa SMD, Thulesius O. Cooling is a potent vasodilator of deep vessels in the rat. Canadian Journal of Physiology and Pharmacology 2001; 79: 899-904.
22. Diao C, Zhu L, Wang H. Cooling and rewarming for brain ischemia or injury: theoretical analysis. Annals of Biomedical Engineering 2003; 31: 346-353.

23. Maloney SK, Mitchell G. Selective brain cooling: role of angularis oculi vein and nasal thermoreception. American Journal of Physiology 1997; 273: R1108-R1116.
24. Nagasaka T, Brinnel H, Hales JR, Ogawa T. Selective brain cooling in hyperthermia: the mechanisms and medical implications. Medical Hypotheses 1998; 50: 203-211.
25. Andrews PJD, Harris B, Murray GD. Randomized controlled trial of effects of the airflow through the upper respiratory tract of intubated brain-injured patients on brain temperature and selective brain cooling. British Journal of Anaesthesia 2005; 94: 330-335.
26. Harris BA, Andrews PJD, Murray GM. Enhanced upper respiratory tract airflow and head fanning reduce brain temperature, without selective brain cooling, in brain-injured, mechanically ventilated patients: A randomized, crossover, factorial trial. British Journal of Anaesthesia 2007; 98: 93-9.
27. Cabanac M, White M. Heat loss from the upper airways and selective brain cooling in humans. Annals of the New York Academy of Sciences 1997; 813: 613-616.
28. Cabanac M. Selective brain cooling and thermoregulatory set-point. Journal of Basic & Clinical Physiology & Pharmacology 1998; 9: 3-13.
29. Gomis P, Rousseaux P, Jolly D, Graftieaux JP. Initial prognostic factors of aneurysmal subarachnoid hemorrhages. Neurochirurgie 1994; 40: 18-30.
30. Rousseaux P, Gomis P, Bazin A, *et al*. Aneurysmal subarachnoid hemorrhage with and without nimodipine. A comparative study with an analysis of the temperature curve. Neurochirurgie 1993; 39: 157-165.
31. Takagi K, Fujimaki T, Kammersgaard LP, Olsen T. Does admission body temperature predict mortality after acute stroke? Stroke 2003; 34: 5-6.
32. Kammersgaard LP, Jorgensen HS, Rungby JA, *et al*. Admission body temperature predicts long-term mortality after acute stroke: The Copenhagen Stroke Study. Stroke 2002; 33: 1759-1762.
33. Dippel DW, van Breda EJ, van Gemert HM, *et al*. Effect of paracetamol (acetaminophen) on body temperature in acute ischemic stroke: a double-blind, randomized phase II clinical trial. Stroke 2001; 32: 1607-1612.
34. Dippel DW, van Breda EJ, van der Worp HB, *et al*. Timing of the effect of acetaminophen on body temperature in patients with acute ischemic stroke. Neurology 2001; 61: 677-679.
35. Hajat C, Hajat S, Sharma P. Effects of poststroke pyrexia on stroke outcome: A meta-analysis of studies in patients. Stroke 2000; 31: 410-414.

36. Reith J, Jorgensen HS, Pedersen PM, *et al*. Body temperature in acute stroke: relation to stroke severity, infarct size, mortality, and outcome. Lancet 1996; 347: 422-425.

9: Musculoskeletal disorders in ICU

DR JOHN MOORE and DR DANIEL CONWAY

Introduction
Musculoskeletal disorders are frequently associated with critical illness. The clinical manifestations are severe with weakness, paresis and difficulty weaning from mechanical ventilation; this leads to extended intensive care unit (ICU) and hospital stays. The pathophysiology of critical illness polyneuropathy and myopathy is multifactorial. Symptoms and signs persist for a prolonged period following ICU discharge and there is emerging evidence to suggest that reducing risk factors during ICU stay and promoting rehabilitation can lead to improved patient outcomes.

Critical Care Polyneuropathy
The term 'critical illness polyneuropathy' (CIP) was first used by Bolton and Zochodne in 1987 [1]. They recognised as others had before them that critically ill patients develop a distinct polyneuropathy characterised by severe weakness, reduced or absent limb reflexes, marked muscle wasting which frequently results in failure to wean from mechanical ventilation.

The incidence is high with up to 50% of adult ICU patients suffering from the syndrome [2]. This can rise to 70-96% in patients with severe sepsis and / or the systemic inflammatory response syndrome (SIRS). Critically ill children are also prone to the same neuromuscular dysfunction [3]. The process probably begins within the first few days of critical illness but the clinical signs together with electrophysiological abnormalities may persist for many years following ICU discharge [4].

Pathophysiology
Critical illness polyneuropathy is an acute axonal sensory-motor polyneuropathy. The precise aetiology and pathogenesis remains unclear but extensive investigation suggests multifactorial causes. In most studies critical illness polyneuropathy is associated with sepsis and / or the systemic inflammatory response syndrome [2] and has led some to postulate that inflammatory cytokines such as tumour necrosis factor, interleukins, histamine, arachidonic acid metabolites and local free radicals might be responsible. Hund's isolation of a serum 3 KDa neurotoxic factor and the elevated immunological G antibody levels (against GM1-ganglioside) in patients with critical

illness polyneuropathy does suggest an immunological aetiology [5, 6].

Thus critical illness polyneuropathy might represent the peripheral neurological manifestations of multiple organ dysfunction. However, biopsies have failed to demonstrate the microvascular changes (such as inflammation, thrombosis, and oxidant injury), that might be expected if this were the case. Also critical illness polyneuropathy does not develop exclusively in patients with sepsis or the systemic inflammatory response syndrome but has been reported in patients with primary respiratory failure [7].

Other causative factors for critical illness polyneuropathy include steroids (associated with thick filament myopathy) and neuromuscular blocking agents. There is some work supporting an association of critical illness polyneuropathy with the use of aminoglycoside antibiotics, total parenteral nutrition and vasopressors [8, 9]. However, this may simply reflect the severity and duration of sepsis and / or the systemic inflammatory response syndrome rather than a direct causative role for these agents.

Diagnosis
Patients are generally diagnosed clinically without formal investigation. Flaccid tetraparesis in combination with reduced or absent reflexes with relative preservation of the cranial nerves is usually found. However, the presence of normal reflexes does not preclude the diagnosis. In less severe forms, the proximal muscles may be spared. The sensory component is a variable alteration in light touch and pin prick sensation.

Electrophysiological features
Electrophysiological studies classically reveal a relatively pure axonal neuropathy. Examination by nerve conduction studies and electromyography quantifies disease severity. Nerve studies of peripheral motor and sensory nerves reveal reduced amplitude of compound action potentials with preservation of conduction velocity. Motor nerves are more affected by critical illness polyneuropathy and patients may have markedly reduced muscle action with normal sensory amplitudes [2, 10]. In these patients, it is important to distinguish them from those with altered neuromuscular transmission or myopathy. Surrounding tissue oedema can disturb the sensory compound potential.

Electromyography shows denervation with fibrillation potentials and positive sharp waves. Although cranial nerves appear clinically to be spared from critical illness polyneuropathy, electrophysiological testing can demonstrate a degree of denervation in these nerves.

Differential Diagnosis
The approach to muscle weakness in intensive care needs to be systematic, so that any reversible pathology is identified. Patients fall into two groups; in one, paralysis develops before ICU admission and in the second after admission. Weakness developing in patients admitted to ICU may well be missed because of the need to stabilise their other systems, or otherwise be attributed to an alternative cause such as septic encephalopathy. Primary brain and spinal cord injury resulting from trauma, infection, vascular insufficiency or neoplasm are usually obvious. However an acute polyneuropathy (such as Guillain-Barre syndrome and porphyria), worsening of a chronic polyneuropathic state (e.g. diabetes mellitus), disease at the neuromuscular junction (e.g. myasthenia gravis) or motor neurone disease need to be considered.

Patients developing peripheral weakness following their ICU admission are most likely to suffer critical illness polyneuropathy and critical illness myopathy. Myelopathy affecting mainly anterior horn cells may result from cardiac arrest, atherosclerosis or surgery on the aorta or severe pulmonary disease. Also disordered neuromuscular transmission from prolonged pharmacological blockade may complicate the clinical picture.

Prognosis and Time Course
Recovery from mild or moderate critical illness polyneuropathy has been previously considered rapid and complete once the initiating insult (e.g. sepsis) has been successfully treated. However in practice, recovery may range from weeks to months with large inter-patient variability. Critical illness polyneuropathy in survivors contributes to increased morbidity and mortality rate when compared to non-affected patients [8, 11]. Garnacho-Montero *et al* performed a prospective study of critically ill septic patients who were mechanically ventilated for more than 7 days looking at critical illness polyneuropathy and its effect on hospital length of stay and mortality. They demonstrated that critical illness polyneuropathy significantly prolonged duration of mechanical ventilation (median 34 days versus 14 days, $p<0.001$) and length of time in hospital (85 days versus 33 days, $p<0.001$). Moreover after adjustment for other variables, critical illness polyneuropathy was the only independent risk factor for weaning failure, increasing the risk by 15 times [11].

In a recent study of long-term survivors of prolonged critical illness, Fletcher *et al* demonstrated neurophysiological abnormalities in over 90% of patients at 5 years, with clinical weakness still present 4 years after ICU discharge [4]. Others report persistent quadriplegia in 32% of the most severely affected individuals and poor quality of life in patients with persisting deficits [12,13].

Treatment and Prevention
As sepsis and / or the systemic inflammatory response syndrome are important aetiological factors in the pathogenesis of critical illness polyneuropathy, possible prevention and limitation relies upon successful and urgent treatment. Previous studies have suggested that when critical illness polyneuropathy is mild or moderate, a faster and more complete recovery can be expected. Trials of immunomodulatory therapies including immunoglobulins have not proved useful at countering critical illness polyneuropathy. However the tight control of blood glucose (between 4.4 and 6.1 mmol/l) achieved in ICU patients by van de Berghe had as a secondary effect a 44% reduction (51.9% conventional treatment group versus 28.7% in the intensive glucose treatment group) in the incidence of critical illness polyneuropathy [14].

Other suggested preventive measures include minimising the use of corticosteroids and neuromuscular blocking agents, although these are probably more useful in avoiding myopathy. This introduces a paradox for corticosteroid administration in treating sepsis and the adult respiratory distress syndrome. It will be interesting to see if other recently introduced sepsis specific therapies, including activated Protein C, have the potential to modulate the critical illness polyneuropathy process.

More general and practical measures for patients with critical illness polyneuropathy include patient and family education about the condition with effective psychological support. The patient requires prolonged intensive and continued physiotherapy as part of their rehabilitation.

Critical Illness Myopathy
Critical illness myopathy (CIM) is an acute primary myopathy characterised by weakness and fatigue in critically ill patients. These clinical features are usually mild but critical illness myopathy often accompanies critical illness polyneuropathy causing paralysis and failure to wean from ventilatory support.

Pathophysiology

Histological examination of patients' muscles with suspected critical illness myopathy shows three main patterns of myopathic changes: necrotising myopathy, myopathy with predominant loss of myosin and a non-specific diffuse non-necrotising myopathy. The exact mechanisms remain the subject of investigation. Whilst immobility and substrate deficiency may account for some muscle loss, they are not sufficient to explain muscle proteolysis seen in severe sepsis. Epidemiological evidence suggests corticosteroid administration, neuromuscular blockade, poor glycaemic control, sepsis and mediators of the systemic inflammatory response play an important role. Using experimental models of critical illness with denervated rat muscle, research groups have demonstrated that muscle will become less excitable. Rich *et al* investigated the effect of steroids and found reduced muscle resting potential with altered Na^+ channels in animal models [15]. The most important change was hyperpolarisation of the voltage dependent Na^+ channels. Depolarization of the resting potential also makes a contribution, but does not cause reduced excitability by itself. Friedrich *et al* performed similar experiments on skinned and intact rat muscle fibres exposed to fractionated serum from septic patients and healthy volunteers [16]. They discovered that low molecular weight serum fractions from septic patients significantly reduced membrane excitability and Na^+ channel activity. They also found septic serum fractions interfering with excitation-contraction coupling in sarcoplasmic reticulum.

Thick filament myopathy often develops independently of critical illness polyneuropathy and is associated with use of steroids and non-depolarising muscle relaxants. Muscle biopsy reveals a selective loss of myosin filaments with other proteins largely unaffected. The reversibility of these changes has been demonstrated experimentally in animal tissue exposed to high dose steroids [17]. Muscle biopsy in necrotising myopathy shows phagocytosis and vacuolisation in conjunction with necrosis of muscle fibres. Unlike other histological types of critical illness myopathy, these features are often accompanied by a rise in serum creatine kinase.

The prevalence of critical illness myopathy in the critically ill population is unknown and will depend upon the case-mix of individual units. In patients with the adult respiratory distress syndrome, the prevalence of critical illness polyneuropathy / critical illness myopathy may be over 50% [18].

Diagnosis

Diagnosing critical illness myopathy, and differentiating critical illness myopathy from critical illness polyneuropathy can be difficult. The clinical features are similar with weakness, a flaccid paralysis and failure to wean from mechanical ventilation. In sedated or uncooperative patients accurate examination of sensory and motor function is difficult and needle electromyography can be misleading. Electrodiagnostics frequently reveal signs such as low amplitude compound muscle action potential, fibrillation potentials and positive spike waves. Unfortunately all of these fail to differentiate critical illness polyneuropathy from critical illness myopathy. Serum creatine kinase is often normal in patients with myopathic changes at muscle biopsy. The diagnostic gold standard for critical illness myopathy remains the muscle biopsy. Unfortunately, this procedure is invasive with delays in obtaining results and it is not part of routine practice. Diagnostic tests which may avoid a biopsy include direct muscle stimulation and then measuring the ratios of nerve:muscle evoked action potential amplitudes. Theoretically patients with critical illness myopathy will have reduced nerve and muscle action potential amplitudes whereas those with critical illness polyneuropathy will have reduced nerve action potential amplitude but normal directly stimulated muscle action potential amplitudes (Figure 1). However this test will not quantify the loss of contractile proteins and is technically challenging to perform. Minimally invasive muscle biopsy has been attempted with actin:myosin ratios proposed as a rapid surrogate marker of critical illness myopathy, where myosin loss predominates [19].

No specific therapies for critical illness myopathy have been identified. Avoiding risk factors and structured rehabilitation remains the mainstay of therapy. As with critical illness polyneuropathy, it is likely that critical illness myopathy will contribute to prolonged ICU and hospital stay. Weakness remains a key feature of recovery from critical care many years after ICU discharge.

Joint and skeletal abnormalities

It is now well established that bone turnover in patients with prolonged critical illness becomes significantly altered [20]. Both osteoblast and osteoclast activity is increased, although osteoblasts tend to be more immature leading to abnormal bone matrix and proportionately greater bone resorption. This can be measured by the elevated serum markers of osteoclast / bone resorption activity such as ß-carboxy terminal cross-linked telopeptide of type I collagen (ß-CTX) in plasma and collagen cross-links in urine [21]. This process

CRITICAL CARE FOCUS 14: UPDATES

Figure 1. Nerve stimulation and direct muscle stimulation. The electromyograph can be obtained from functional muscle which has lost adequate nerve supply, thus differentiating between myopathy and neuropathy. Modified from Latronico [26].

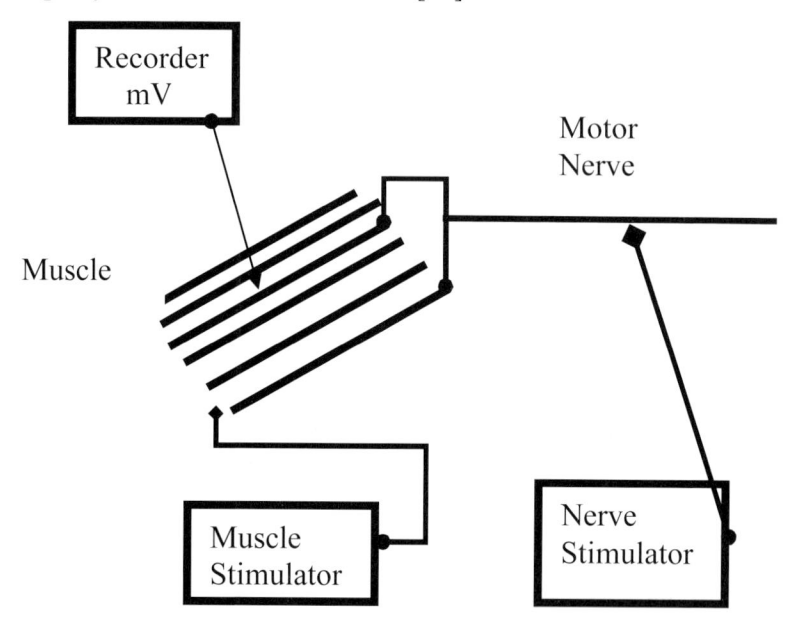

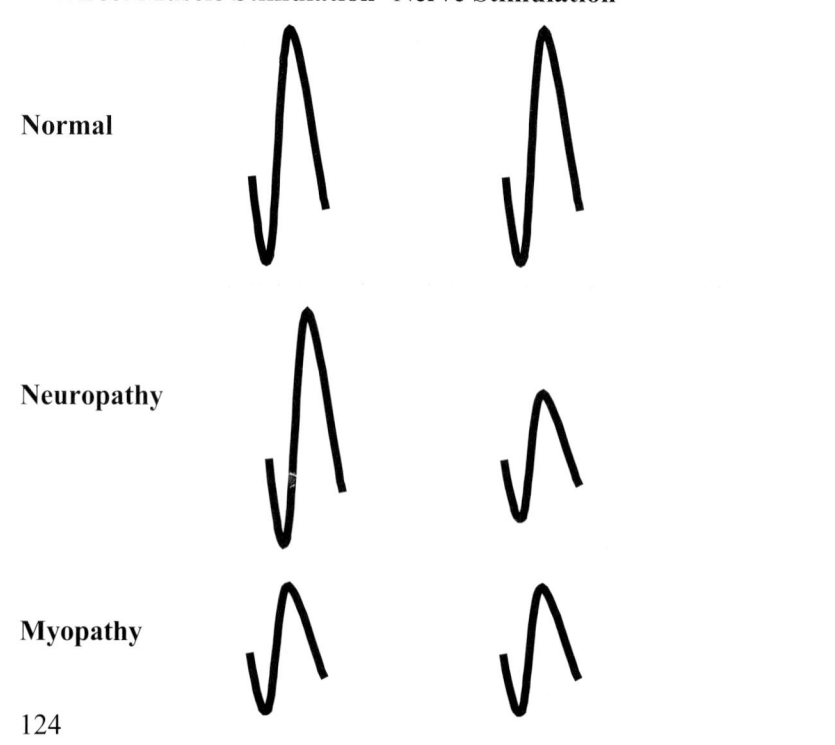

of increased bone resorption probably predisposes towards osteoporosis and altered fracture healing.

The mechanisms responsible are likely to be a disturbance of the normal homeostatic endocrine and immune functions, with additional contributions from immobilisation, nutritional deficiency especially calcium and vitamins, and cytokine activation [20, 21]. Bone markers of resorption are highest in those patients with sepsis, although surprisingly have not correlated with interleukin-6, interleukin-1 or tumour necrosis factor-a levels. Specific endocrine disturbances suggested as causative include hyperparathyroidism, renal insufficiency, hypogonadism, raised cortisol levels, secondary hypothyroidism and possibly most importantly vitamin D deficiency. Van de Berghe *et al.* attempted to normalise vitamin D levels in critically ill patients, as part of their assessment of bone remodelling [21]. Despite high dose supplementation, they were unable to reach normal vitamin D levels and so could not comment upon any beneficial effect in terms of reduced bone resorption.

Improving Outcomes from Musculoskeletal Dysfunction following Critical Illness

The musculoskeletal system is designed to keep moving. Muscle bulk reduces rapidly with immobility and with critical illness polyneuropathy and critical illness myopathy, massive muscle loss (2% of muscle mass per day, up to 50% of total muscle mass) can take place. Weakness and fatigue are common challenges faced by patients recovering from critical illness. Patients are also at significant risk of contractures particularly of the shoulders, hands, hips and ankles. Early mobilisation is crucial, even when the patient is intubated and ventilated. Hoists, walking aids and splints all help rehabilitation.

Weakness will be exacerbated by poor nutritional state, mood disturbance, pain and cognitive impairment. Treating musculoskeletal problems involves reducing the factors thought to cause critical illness polyneuropathy and / or critical illness myopathy followed by a structured rehabilitation programme tailored to reverse muscle and nerve loss.

Minimising risk factors for critical illness polyneuropathy and / or critical illness myopathy requires foresight and vigilance as symptoms usually become apparent during weaning long after the patient has been exposed to the cause(s). A balance is often required. For example, physiological replacement for adrenocortical dysfunction in septic shock has been shown to improve outcome for patients but has not been associated with critical illness polyneuropathy nor myopathy.

CRITICAL CARE FOCUS 14: UPDATES

High dose corticosteroid administration for severe adult respiratory distress syndrome improves oxygenation but not hospital survival. Complications of high dose steroids such as gastrointestinal haemorrhage, infection and critical illness polyneuropathy and myopathy may account for the lack of benefit of steroid therapy despite improvements in respiratory function [22].

Ideally the rehabilitation process should begin whilst the patient is in the critical care unit. Traditionally physiotherapy on ICU has focussed on clearing secretions and improving respiratory function. A more comprehensive approach to whole-body rehabilitation will improve physical and respiratory recovery. A report from a ventilation rehabilitation unit which offers all patients a structured, gym-based physiotherapist-led rehabilitation programme suggests that improvements in limb and trunk strength and fatigability occurred in tandem with improvements in ventilation to the point where all patients were successfully weaned from long term ventilatory support [23]. Dysphagia has been reported in over 50% of patients ventilated for greater than 24 hours. Changes in swallowing can be subtle with silent aspiration a common finding. Routine endoscopic evaluation of swallow has not been shown to reduce the incidence of aspiration pneumonia [24]. Bedside screening of swallowing function in patients with tracheostomies using blue dye-stained water will identify patients at risk of difficulties in swallowing.

The period following discharge from critical care areas can be challenging for patients and carers as the surroundings are unfamiliar, with less monitoring and lower staffing levels. Discovery interviews of ICU survivors have identified this period as a major source of stress and it has been termed 'transfer anxiety'. This can lead to a hiatus in rehabilitation as a period of adjustment takes place. Many hospitals now operate an ICU outreach service which can bridge the gap between critical care and the general wards with the intention of reducing mortality, re-admission to ICU and promoting physical and psychological recovery. Follow-up teams are multi-disciplinary with input from doctors, nurses, physiotherapists, speech therapists, psychologists and occupational therapists. Collaboration allows a co-ordinated approach to rehabilitation whilst maintaining close links with critical care.

The value of this type of multi-disciplinary approach to recovery has been demonstrated by Jones *et al.* in three UK hospitals in a randomised controlled trial [25]. They allocated ICU survivors to receive routine follow-up care with ward visits and an out-patient clinic or routine care with a self-help manual. The self-help package was based on similar work in cardiac and pulmonary rehabilitation. It included information and practical advice regarding nutrition, smoking cessation and dealing with psychological problems such as panic attacks, phobias, anxiety and depression. The intervention group also received a graded six week exercise plan. The heterogeneous nature of critically ill patients following discharge means that a single set of exercises will not suit all patients. The manual used the Borg Ratings of Perceived Exertion Scale to allow patients to progress through the physical rehabilitation according to their individual needs. This process was further enhanced by input from physiotherapists suggesting appropriate exercises. The study recorded a number of standardised measurements for psychological morbidity and quality of life. The physical function domains of the Short Form 36 (SF 36) Quality of Life Questionnaire were the primary outcome measures for physical recovery. This was measured at two and six months from the start of rehabilitation. At both these time points the intervention group using the manuals demonstrated significantly higher physical function scores than patients receiving routine care (intervention group scored closer to normal at 8 weeks and at 6 months, p=0.006). ICU follow-up services have responded to this encouraging research by implementing self-help manuals, physiotherapist-led rehabilitation and exercise programmes for patients discharged from critical care.

Conclusion

Musculoskeletal dysfunction as a consequence of critical illness is an independent risk factor for prolonged hospital stay and mortality. Patients with severe sepsis, immobility, poor nutrition and administration of drugs such as muscle relaxants and high dose corticosteroids are at increased risk of developing critical illness polyneuropathy and / or myopathy. No specific treatments exist but optimal glycaemic control and minimising exposure to risk factors should be considered. Following critical illness, there is evidence to support multidisciplinary rehabilitation programmes in order to improve quality of life outcomes for patients.

References

1. Zochodne DW, Bolton CF, Wells GA, *et al.* Critical illness polyneuropathy. A complication of sepsis and multiple organ failure. Brain 1987; 110: 819-842.
2. Bolton CF. Sepsis and the systemic inflammatory response syndrome: neuromuscular manifestations. Critical Care Medicine 1996; 24: 1408-1416.
3. Sheth RD, Bolton CF. Neuromuscular complications of sepsis in children. Journal of Child Neurology 1995; 10: 346-352.

4   Fletcher SN, Kennedy DD, Ghosh IR, *et al.* Persistent neuromuscular and neurophysiologic abnormalities in long-term survivors of prolonged critical illness. Critical Care Medicine 2003; 31: 1012-1016.
5   Hund E, Herbert M, Becker CM, Hacke W. A humoral neurotoxic factor in sera of patients with critical illness polyneuropathy. Critical Care Medicine 1996; 24: 1328-1333.
6   Terasako K, Seo N, Murayama T, Kai T, Hirata S, Fujiwara T. Are autoimmune mechanisms involved in critical illness polyneuropathy? Intensive Care Medicine 1995; 21: 96-97.
7   Gorson KC, Ropper AH. Acute respiratory failure neuropathy: A variant of critical illness neuropathy. Critical Care Medicine 1993; 21: 267-271.
8   Leijten FS, De Weerd AW, Poortvliet DC, De Ridder VA, Ulrich C, Harink-De Weerd JE. Critical illness polyneuropathy in multiple organ dysfunction syndrome and weaning from the ventilator. Intensive Care Medicine 1996; 22: 856-861.
9   Waldhausen E, Mingers B, Lippers P, Keser G. Critical illness polyneuropathy due to parenteral nutrition. Intensive Care Medicine 1997; 23: 922-923.
10 Hund E, Genzwurker H, Bohrer H, Jakob H, Thiele R, Hacke W. Predominant involvement of motor fibres in patients with critical illness polyneuropathy. British Journal of Anaesthesia 1997; 78: 274-78.
11 Garnacho-Montero J, Amaya-Villar R, Garcia-Garmendia JL, Madrazo-Osuna J, Ortiz-Leyba C. Effect of critical illness polyneuropathy on the withdrawal from mechanical ventilation and the length of stay in septic patients. Critical Care Medicine 2005; 33: 349-354.
12 de Seze M, Petit H, Wiart L, *et al.* Critical illness polyneuropathy. A 2 year follow-up study in 19 severe cases. European Neurology 2000; 43: 61-69.
13 Zifko UA. Long-term outcome of critical illness polyneuropathy. Muscle Nerve 2000; 52: 49-52.
14 van den Berghe G, Wouters P, Weekers F, *et al.* Intensive insulin therapy in the critically ill patients. New England Journal of Medicine 2001; 345: 1359-1367.
15 Rich MM, Pinter MJ. Crucial role of sodium channel fast inactivation in muscle fibre inexcitability in a rat model of critical illness myopathy. Journal of Physiology 2003; 547: 555-566.
16 Friedrich O, Hund E, Weber C, Hacke W, Fink RH. Critical illness myopathy serum fractions affect membrane excitability and intracellular calcium release in mammalian skeletal muscle. Journal of Neurology 2004; 251: 53-65.

17 Massa R, Carpenter S, Holland P, Karpati G. Loss and renewal of thick myofilaments in glucocorticoid-treated rat soleus after denervation and reinnervation. Muscle Nerve 1992; 15: 1290-1298.
18 Bercker S, Weber-Carstens S, Deja M, *et al.* Critical illness polyneuropathy and myopathy in patients with acute respiratory distress syndrome. Critical Care Medicine 2005; 33: 711-715.
19 Stibler H, Edstrom L, Ahlbeck K, Remahl S, Ansved T. Electrophoretic determination of the myosin/actin ratio in the diagnosis of critical illness myopathy. Intensive Care Medicine 2003; 29: 1515-1527.
20 Nierman DM, Mechanick JI. Bone hyperresorption is prevalent in chronically critically ill patients. Chest 1998; 114: 1122-1128.
21 Van den Berghe G, Van Roosbroeck D, Vanhove P, Wouters PJ, De Pourcq L, Bouillon R. Bone turnover in prolonged critical illness: effect of vitamin D. Journal of Clinical Endocrinology and Metabolism 2003; 88: 4623-4632.
22 Steinberg KP, Hudson LD, Goodman RB, *et al.* National Heart, Lung and Blood Institute Acute Respiratory Distress Syndrome (ARDS) Clinical Trials Network. Efficacy and safety of corticosteroids for persistent acute respiratory distress syndrome. New England Journal of Medicine 2006; 354: 1671-1684.
23 Martin UJ, Hincapie L, Nimchuk M, Gaughan J, Criner GJ. Impact of whole-body rehabilitation in patients receiving chronic mechanical ventilation. Critical Care Medicine 2005; 33: 2259-2265.
24 Barquist E, Brown M, Cohn S, Lundy D, Jackowski J. Postextubation fiberoptic endoscopic evaluation of swallowing after prolonged endotracheal intubation: a randomized, prospective trial. Critical Care Medicine 2001; 29: 1710-1713.
25 Jones C, Skirrow P, Griffiths RD, *et al.* Rehabilitation after critical illness. A randomised controlled trial. Critical Care Medicine 2003; 31: 2456-2461.
26 Latronico N, Peli E, Botteri M. Critical illness myopathy and neuropathy. Current Opinion in Critical Care 2005; 11: 126-132.

10: The London Bombings, July 7th 2005

DR HUGH MONTGOMERY

Explosive Devices
When explosive material detonates, a large volume of gas is very rapidly generated. A high-pressure blast wave expands outwards at the speed of sound causing *primary* injuries (mainly at air interfaces such as the lung, ear and bowel). Mass gas/air movement ('blast wind') then carries solid matter into the patient (*secondary* injury), or hurls the patient into surrounding infrastructure (which, with direct disruptive effects, constitute *tertiary* injury). Heat, flame and inhalation of hot gases and smoke cause *quaternary* injuries. Confined spaces worsen the biological impact of such devices [1]: surface reflections amplify and prolong the blast wave, prevent dissipation of heat and smoke and channel blast wind. Unfortunately, the UK mainland, and London in particular, has witnessed a large number of terrorist explosions.

Terrorism in London
Mainland Britain has been the target of numerous terrorist attacks throughout its modern history. The 19th Century Fenians (Fianna were legendary Irish Warriors) launched their first bomb attack in Clerkenwell, London in 1867, when their attempt to free two members from jail resulted in 138 casualties of whom 8.7% died. Their campaign continued and in 1883, they threatened to blow a Scotland Yard Superintendent 'off his stool' and also to attack public buildings in London. At 21.00 hrs on the 30th May, an empty building at the centre of Great Scotland Yard was indeed bombed. The device was left in a cast iron urinal; fortunately the only casualty was a cabbie injured by flying glass. Bombs also exploded in the Carlton Club and outside the home of Sir Watkin Wynne (an aristocrat of a famous Welsh borders family), whilst a device left beneath Nelson's Column failed to detonate. The following year, bombs also damaged London Bridge, the Tower of London and the House of Commons.

In the 20th Century, the increased terrorist activity of the Irish Republican Army (IRA) peaked between 1969 and 2000. In 1972 alone, the UK witnessed 1500 separate bombings causing 5005 casualties. Many of these attacks are well remembered: the Harrod's bomb, 17th December 1983 (85 casualties of which 5 died), the Warrington bombs, 20th March 1993 (two devices causing 58 casualties, of which two children died), Horseguards' Parade, 19th

July 1982 (25 casualties of which 8 died), Regent's Park Bandstand, 19th July 1982 (30 casualties of which 6 died) and Victoria Station, 18th February 1991 (41 casualties with one death).

In the 1990s, attacks were more often targeted at commercial property or transport infrastructure: August 1991 (three incendiary devices found beneath a train at Hammersmith Station), December 1991 (a bomb exploded on a railway line near Clapham Junction), December 1991 (a device exploded on an underground train at Neasden Underground Depot), December 1991 (an explosion on an underground train at Harrow on the Hill), January 1992 (an incendiary device discovered under a seat of a train at Elephant and Castle), February 1992 (an incendiary device failed to explode on a train at Neasden), February 1992 (an incendiary ignited on a train at Barking Underground) and April 1993 and February 1995, when financial targets in the City of London and Canary Wharf were respectively bombed. While there was no major loss of life, civilians were injured (as in the explosion at a toilet at London Bridge Station in February 1992, when 29 people were injured).

More recently, the lone disgruntled individual, facilitated by the increased accessibility of information on the world-wide web, poses a new risk. On 30th April 1999, such an individual exploded a home-made device in a Soho pub, killing three people and injuring more than 80. This was one of three attacks by the same individual; the others were in Brixton (39 injured but no deaths) and Brick Lane (only six injured, after a passer-by drove the device away in the boot of his car).

Against this background, the London attacks of 7th July 2005 represent a substantial new direction in both scale and *modus operandi*. These attacks were orchestrated by a remote international terrorist organisation and utilised local (English) citizens. Civilians were again targeted and for the first time suicide bombing was a feature.

The July 7th Bombs
At approximately 08.50 hrs on that Thursday morning, three independent bombs were detonated within 50 seconds of each other on the London Underground Network.

Between Kings Cross and Russell Square Underground Stations, a device exploded in the front carriage of Train 311, one minute after leaving Kings Cross Station and travelling 450 m. The explosion

CRITICAL CARE FOCUS 14: UPDATES

occurred near the back of the first carriage also causing severe damage to the front of carriage number two. Staff from the neighbouring National Hospital for Neurology and Neurosurgery and Great Ormond Street Hospital for Sick Children responded rapidly to assist paramedic ambulance crews. Twenty-five individuals died at the scene. Many 'walking wounded' were treated at the scene but 236 individuals (including 36 severely injured victims) were taken to local hospitals. Two adults were admitted to the Children's Intensive Care Unit.

Only 100 m from the end of the station platform at Edgware Road, another device exploded on Train 216, eight minutes after leaving Kings Cross Station, and just after it had left Edgware Road. This explosion killed seven at the scene. Within three hours, 80 other victims had been triaged at the scene, and St Mary's Hospital had received over 38 casualties, 24 of whom were in a critical or serious condition.

Meanwhile, 200 m from the platform end at Aldgate Station, a device exploded on the floor of the third carriage of Train 204, eight minutes after it had left Kings Cross Station. The carriage was 90 m into the tunnel from Liverpool Street Station. Seven victims died at the scene, with more than 100 wounded (16 severely). Patients were triaged and transported (by ambulance and three buses) to the Royal London Hospital, which received 208 casualties from this and other sites. Overall, 27 patients were admitted.

It took some time to recognise the nature of these attacks. A Code Amber call (requiring all passengers to be immediately taken off trains at stations and moved above ground) was issued at 09.18.

Meanwhile, the number 55 bus was travelling from Hackney Wick to Marble Arch, where it turned around at 09.00 hrs for its return journey. It reached Euston at 09:35 hrs, where those evacuated from the tube stations boarded. One of the evacuees included the next suicide bomber, who had been unable to gain entry to a Northern line train before his colleague's bombs exploded. The bus was diverted from its normal route because of road closures in the Kings Cross area (due to the earlier tube bombings). At 09.47 hrs, a device exploded near the back of the upper deck at Tavistock Square junction with Upper Woburn Place. Fourteen doctors, many from the nearby British Medical Association, gave immediate assistance. Thirteen individuals died at the scene. Most of the passengers at the front of the top and lower decks survived whereas those at the top and bottom rear bore the brunt of the explosion.

THE LONDON BOMBINGS

Overall, four suicide bombers injured 650 people of whom 45 were critically or seriously injured. Three hundred and fifty were treated at the scenes; the Royal London Hospital received 208 casualties, the highest number presenting to a single institution. One hundred were hospitalised overnight. By morning, 22 of these remained in 'serious or critical' conditions and one person subsequently died. Overall, 56 people died in the four bombs giving a mortality rate of 8%. This mortality rate was almost identical to that in Madrid in March 2004, when 191(or 8.4%) of the 2253 injured died [2]. In both Madrid and London, most who died perished at the scene.

These mortality rates seem remarkably consistent for terrorist attacks: for example, 8.7% of the victims of the 1867 Clerkenwell bomb died. Mortality rates are usually determined by the size of blast relative to its confines and the proximity of potential casualties. Thus, mortality may be lower where explosions occur in open spaces (e.g. Victoria Station 2.4%, Warrington 3.4%), but will be higher where large blasts occur close to multiple individuals (Regent's Park Bandstand 20%).

The parallels between London and Madrid (i.e. many casualties, higher mortality and severe injuries) reflect the site and timing of attacks. The confined areas in which explosions occurred increased the casualty (and mortality) rates. Indeed, the mortality rates at the different sites in London on 7th July also reflect differences in the environments in which the explosions occurred. The Circle line runs 7 m beneath the surface and is fairly wide with twin tracks allowing blast (and heat) dissipation in the Edgware Road explosion. Thus, St. Mary's Hospital saw only 38 injured with seven deaths. On the other hand, the Piccadilly Line (the Kings Cross/ Russell Square explosion) is up to 30 m beneath ground with single track and narrow (15 cm) clearance to the tunnel wall. In this explosion, more than 260 were injured, of whom 25 (9.6%) died.

Problems in Immediate Management

The simultaneous detonation of multiple devices throughout an underground transport network causes numerous logistic problems. All transport infrastructure grinds to a halt, preventing movement of emergency personnel to their places of work and access of those on duty to the injured. Once on-scene, access to the train carriages proved difficult; the temperatures in the Piccadilly Line ultimately reached 60°C (140°F) and the single-line tunnel site limited access.

CRITICAL CARE FOCUS 14: UPDATES

Meanwhile, demands were high: over 100 ambulances (and more than 250 staff) were deployed by the London Ambulance Service. Communications proved difficult: the mobile telephone networks soon became overloaded by civilian use, preventing adequate communication between hospitals and sites of explosion.

Meanwhile, hospitals also faced their own pressures. The management of mass casualties requires large numbers of staff, and the rapid formation of numerous 'sub-teams'. The unique mechanisms of explosive injury, and the combinations of primary, secondary, tertiary and quaternary injuries, is not encountered in any other situation [3]. Such clinical presentations will be unfamiliar to most healthcare staff. Demands for equipment are high and extra capacity is urgently required in operating theatres and intensive care units (ICUs). All supporting services ranging from catering to switchboards, laundry to laboratories will be under intense pressure. Re-stocking and re-supply can be impossible without an effective transport system. Some staff are likely to be 'off post' and contacting a colleague can prove difficult when mobile telephones do not work. All of these problems are compounded by difficulties in maintaining the 'chain of forensic evidence'.

Demands on hospital beds can be high. Survivors once moved from ICU may require prolonged hospital care for many weeks or months. Ill health and the demand for treatment do not cease; a brief audit in London after 7th July found more remote hospitals loaded with 'routine emergencies' that day which blocked beds for elective work for many subsequent days and weeks. This had financial as well as social repercussions: people had to travel across London to visit hospitalised family members.

Specific Problems for Intensive Care
ICUs face major demands at such times. ICU bed availability is usually limited as may be the availability of trained staff, especially if commuting is disrupted. Furthermore, generic ICU skills are in demand in mass casualty situations for management of major injuries, or provision of vascular access, airway support or mechanical ventilation. Critical care transport requires specialist skills and appropriate equipment. Movement of patients around the hospital is frequent and transfer *between* hospitals common; an influx of critically ill patients will exacerbate these pressures.

Patient identification may be a problem: July 7th bombing injured a deaf/dumb man who was unable to confirm his identify to anyone before the need for intubation arose. It took several days for his relatives to find him in ICU.

Staffing ratios may be inadequate to maintain the required number of Level 1 beds, and fatigue may occur. The diverse nature and site of injuries makes clinical management of bomb victims particularly intensive: return to theatre for plastic or orthopaedic surgical intervention may occur on a daily (or more frequent) basis.

Future Problems and Responses
Further terrorist attacks seem inevitable, and many of the problems identified above may recur. These must be addressed area by area. For example, what has been done to maximise surge capacity or ICU beds? Have robust communication networks (both to, and within, hospitals) been established and tested? What has been done to increase critical care transport provision? Bomb victims need specialist care, such as plastic surgery and this will require the clearing of ICU beds in specialist centres and the transfer of other patients out to other non-specialist hospitals. Other elements may cause added complexity. For example, CBRN (chemical, nuclear, biological, radiological) agents may augment the lethality of conventional devices; Sarin was released into the Tokyo subway system in October 1995.

Planning and rehearsal are needed at every level. Such preparation needs to be at individual, institutional, regional and national levels. Special attention needs to be paid to the points at which other services interface with critical care. Part of the effectiveness of the response to the July 7th bombing was due to recent rehearsal in an all-agency response to a notional explosion in a deep subway tunnel, and regular table top exercises. NHS preparedness is essential and chief executives are legally responsible for planning and practicing for all forms of attack.

Only two weeks after the July 7th bombing, a second series of four explosions occurred on the London Underground. Fortunately, the detonators alone exploded, and there were no serious casualties. This re-inforces the importance of being prepared; unless planning and preparation remain current, London may not be so lucky next time.

Acknowledgements
I thank the following individuals and organisations who willingly offered data: The Metropolitan Police, London Ambulance Service, hospital press offices, members of the UK Intensive Care Society, and the surgeons and physicians at the receiving hospitals. Particular

thanks go to Drs Gareth Davies and David Lockey (Consultants, London Helicopter Emergency Medical Service).

References
1. Chaloner E. Blast Injury in Enclosed Spaces. British Medical Journal 2005; 331: 119-120.
2. Gutierrez de Caballos JP, Turegano Fuentes F, Perez Diaz D, Sanz Sanchez M, Martin Llorente C, Guerrero Sanz JE. Casualties treated at the closest hospital in the Madrid, March 11, terrorist bombings. Critical Care Medicine 2005; 33: S107-S112.
3. Kluger Y, Kashuk J, Mayo A. Terror bombing- mechanisms, consequences and implications. Scandinavian Journal of Surgery 2004; 93: 11-14.

11: Trauma outcome: Is it all in the genes?

PROF PETER V GIANNOUDIS and DR STATHIS KATSOULIS

Introduction
Trauma describes wounds ranging from a little scratch to life threatening multiple injuries. The body counteracts traumatic events with a standard response designed to restore the normal physiological state. Technological advances and shorter rescue times have aided effective resuscitation but the clinical challenges have moved to treatment of the later host response to injury. Trauma patients are at risk of progressive organ dysfunction from what appears to be an uncontrolled immune response. In recent years, better understanding of the pathophysiology of the immune cascade triggered by both traumatic and surgical injury has contributed enormously to knowledge of the aetiology of septic complications and post-traumatic lung injury [1,2]. In some respects, the response to trauma resembles exaggerated activation of the immune system with cell-mediated damage to remote organs while in other respects immunosuppression predominates [3,4]. Many alterations in inflammatory function have been demonstrated both clinically and experimentally within hours of trauma and haemorrhage, suggesting that a cascade of abnormalities leading ultimately to the adult respiratory distress syndrome (ARDS) and multiple organ dysfunction syndrome (MODS) is initiated in the immediate post-injury period [5,6]. Important mediators regulating these events are cytokines. These are synthesized and released in large quantities by leucocytes and endothelial cells after exposure to different chemical and physiological stimuli [7,8]. They mediate a wide array of systemic and local biological functions and so eventually affect patient outcome.

However, some patients appear not to have the expected outcome. Some patients do poorly while others do better than predicted. In the early 1990s it was recognized that this difference in the context of trauma or surgery was the result of biological variation [9]. Such biological variation is highly dependent on the genetic constitution and the importance of genes as cause of diseases or as predisposing factors is now indisputable (Table 1) [10-19]. Polymorphisms (see glossary for definition) are key to this variation. Some are mutations located within endonuclease restriction sites [19-22]. Others are single nucleotide polymorphisms [13,14,18,23,24] or consist of insertions or deletions of larger fragments [16]. The polymorphism can be located within the gene [13,16,23] or in the promoter region

Table 1. The association between genes, alleles, polymorphisms and their effects.

GENES	ALLELES - POLYMORPHISM	CORRELATIONS – EFFECTS
ACE	287-base pair fragment deletion (D)[152]	↑ plasma and tissue ACE activity[152] ↑ D allele in ARDS ↔ mortality[153,203]
apoE	APOe3 allelic variant[184]	↓ incidence of severe sepsis ↓ ICU length of stay[184]
BPI	Lys216Glu	No association noted except for male patients and Cys98Gly allele and ↑susceptibility[116]
CD14	T allele (C→T transition at -159)[124,125,127,126]	sCD14 levels ↔ ↑ mortality in septic shock[124,129,128,125,130,127,126] No association[204]
	159TT genotype of CD14 in promoter[128,114,124]	Susceptibility to and outcome of septic shock[128,124] ↑ positive bacterial cultures on ICU admissions[114] genetic risk factor for death from septic shock[128,124]
Factor V Leiden	506 Arg→Gln in exon[146]	Lower 28-day mortality, lesser vasopressor use at baseline in heterozygotes[146]
HSP (HSP70 familly) HSPA1A HSPA1B HSPA1L	Gen. Polym. of HSP70 genes[205] HSPA1-B1267*A genotype[165] HSPA1B1267A>G, HSPA1A-27G>C, HSPA1L2437C>T[166] HSPA1B-179C>T[167]	Not associated with susceptibility or outcome of severe sepsis[205] Greater risk of septic shock[165] Inflammatory and autoimmune diseases[166] Affects HSP70 production, ↑mRNA levels of HSPA1A and HSPA1B determinant of individual susceptibility to infections and

	HSPA1L2437C>T[206]	inflammatory disease[167]
	HSPA1L 1209 C→T exon[205]	↑IL-1 plasma level, ↑liver failure in post-trauma surgery[206]
	HSPA1B 2075 G→A exon[205]	No association with infection susceptibility or survival in septic patients[205]
	HSPA1B A-1538 G promoter[206]	No association with infection susceptibility or survival in septic patients[205]
		↑TNF plasma levels, not associated with outcome in post-trauma surgery patients[206]
IFN-γ R1	AA microsatellite polymorphism[105]	Correlated strongly with infection[105]
IFN-γ	First intron of the IFN-γ gene[100]	Development of sepsis after trauma[100]
	D allele Homozygocity (DD)[100]	↑ chance of sepsis after traumatic injury[100]
	IFN-γ VNTR and IFN γR VNTR[105,100]	Possibly associated with infection risk[105,100]
IL-1Ra	Allele *2 Homozygosity[101,102,44]	6.47-fold increased mortality[101,102] Septic susceptibility, ↑mortality in severe sepsis,[101,102,44] ↑frequency in septic patients[44]
	IL-1Ra A2 allele[101,44,102]	Associated with susceptibility to sepsis[101,44,102]
IL-1a	VNTR 46 base pairs, intron	No association with susceptibility to sepsis[102]
IL-1β	-1903 (T→C) in promotor ↔ endonuclease *AluI*[54,55]	
	-5810 (G→A) in intron 4 ↔ endonuclease *BsoFI*[54,55]	Not associated with outcome after sepsis[44]
	-5887 (C→T) in exon 5 ↔ endonuclease *TaqI*[54,55]	*TaqI*'s 13.4 kb product represents an IL-1β "high-secretor" phenotype[55]
	-511 promoter	↑IL-1β in LPS-stimulated monocytes.[55] Not associated with susceptibility to sepsis[44,102]
IL-6		Susceptibility to sepsis[153], ↑ mortality in severe sepsis[153]

	*Sfa*NI (-174) Homozygosity[64,63] Promoter (-174GC) – C allele[65] G→C at position -174[68]	↓ IL-6; LPS or IL-1 → slight ↑ IL-6 secretion[64,63] ↓ gene promoter activity[65] Adverse outcome in several inflam.diseases[68] unclear association in septic outcome
	Homozygous IL-6 -174G genotype[69] IL-6 174G/C polymorphism[69]	Observed in patients with SIRS[69] Associated with post-SIRS severity[69] improved post-severe sepsis survival when having genotype GG[69,67]
	C/C/G, G/G/G, G/C/C haplotypes[68]	Strongly associated with ↑mortality and organ dysfunction in critically ill patients with SIRS[68]
IL-10	Allele IL10.R3[92] Haplotype IL10.R2/IL10.G14[92] Haplotype IL-10.R3/IL10.G7[92] A allele of the -1082 polymorphism in the IL-10 gene promoter[82] G allele of the -1082 polymorphism in the IL-10 gene promoter[82] Genotype -597AC[91] Genotype -592AC[91,79] IL-10 -1082 allele 1[81] -1082 in the promoter region[81] G-1082A in promoter	IL-10 secretion < any other IL10.R allele[92] Associated with highest IL-10 secretion overall[92] Associated with lowest IL-10 secretion[92] Sepsis susceptibility[82] Higher stimulated IL-10 production[82] ↑ mortality in severe sepsis[82] Higher overall MOD scores[91] Over represented in the MODS group[91] 3.3-fold ↑ in risk of developing MODS[91] ↓levels of IL-10, ↑mortality in sepsis[79] No association in mortality or septic incidence[81] More likely to have severe sepsis[81] Maybe susceptible to severe sepsis[81] No association in IL-10 secretion, sepsis or mortality[79]

IL-18 promoter	-607bp CA genotype combined with -137bp GC genotype (CA/GC)[99]	↑allele frequency in septic patients[80] ↑risk of shock from pneumococcus[80] ↑mortality + ↑illness severity in community-acquired pneumonias[98] 27% of patients developed sepsis[99]
LBP	291 position[117]	↑septic risk in males[116] Not associated with post-trauma sepsis[117]
MBL	52 Arg→Cys (D exon allele)[207,208,209] 54 Gly→Asp (B allele)[207,208,209] 57 Gly→Gly (C allele)[207,208,209]	↓MBL → sepsis, severe sepsis, septic shock[118] ↑susceptibility to bacterial infections[207,208,209] ↑prevalence of positive bact. cultures and sepsis[114] not altered prevalence of septic shock[114], not ↓ 28-day survival.[114]
MIF	G-173C in promoter	↑ frequency of the C allele in sepsis or in sepsis-induced acute lung injury
PAI-1	4G/5G insertion/deletion promoter[134]	Poor septic outcome[134] ↑ cytokines, acute-phase proteins, coagulation parameters[134] Variations in PAI-1 production[134], risk of severe complications, septic mortality[134], ↑PAI-1 levels, worse outcome from sepsis, ↑risk of death[210,211,212,137]
	PAI-1 4G allele[137]	↑ concentrations of PAI-1[137], poor survival rate after severe trauma[137]
SP-B	Intron 4[133]	In ARDS & direct pulmonary injury in females[133]
Tissue Factor	1208 I allele[147]	↑ plasma levels of TF[147] ↑ risk of venous thrombosis[147]
TLR2		↑ prevalence of positive bacterial cultures and sepsis[114] Not altered prevalence of septic shock[114] Not ↓ 28-day survival[114]

	753 Arg→Gln in exon[213,214]	Gram-positive bacterial infections[114] Predisposition to life-threatening bacterial infection[214] No association morbidity/mortality caused by *Staph. aureus*[213,214]
TLR4	TLR4 Asp299Gly allele[110] TLR4Asp299Gly and TLR4Thr399Ile alleles[110] TLR4Thr399Ile alleles[215]	↑ mortality in SIRS, ↑ Gram-negative infections in critically ill patients[108,111] Exclusively in patients with septic shock[110] Higher prevalence of Gram-negative infections[110,108] Hyporesponsiveness to airway LPS[107] Unchanged post-surgical sepsis incidence[215]
TNF	Position –308 of TNF2 allele[30,31] NcoI in the first intron[28] (TNF-b) NcoI[47] TNF-b2/b2 genotype[47] TNFB2 Homozygosity[44,42,45,43] (male septic patients only) TNF-α G-376A promoter[33] TNF-α G-238A promoter[216]	↑ septic shock susceptibility,[33,217] ↑3.7fold risk of death,[33,32,217] ↓outcome in major trauma and ARDS[30,31] ↓ TNF production[28] ↑ mortality in severe sepsis[47] Severe complications and mortality from sepsis[47] ↑ severe sepsis and worse outcome. ↑TNF-α concentrations, ↑MODS scores[44,42,45,43,41] Allele only detected in non-survivors post-septic shock,[33] No difference between severe sepsis and control groups[34] ↑risk of death in community-acquired pneumonia patients[216]
VEGF	CT and TT genotypes[150] T allele in the +936 CT[150]	↑ mean APACHE III score (in ARDS)[150] ↓ VEGF plasma levels[150]

[14,15]. Polymorphisms are based upon different alleles. A specific polymorphic variation can be associated with a genetic disease (such as Sickle Cell Disease, thalassaemia, Huntington's Disease, Duchenne's Muscular Dystrophy, Friedreich's Ataxia, Familial Mediterranean Fever or Crohn's Disease). The polymorphism can also interact with the environment which then can exert detrimental actions. For example carcinogenic substances such as tobacco and industrial chemicals, dietary biologically active substances can affect gene transcription.

In the context of this emerging evidence, the currently available literature in terms of genetic predisposition to sepsis following trauma and surgery is reviewed.

Polymorphisms
Genetic polymorphisms related to post-traumatic sepsis have been discovered and investigated at various levels. Their effects in sepsis are described below and can be categorised as altering: i) cytokines, ii) receptors, iii) binding proteins and iv) other inflammation - related proteins.

i) Cytokines
Tumour Necrosis Factor (TNF)
The human TNF locus consists of two tandemly arranged and closely related sequences on the short arm of chromosome 6 which encodes for two cytokines (TNF-a and TNF-ß), using the same surface receptors [25,26]. Wilson *et al.* reported a functional bi-allelic polymorphism (TNF1 and TNF2) in the promoter region of the TNF gene at position –308 [27]. Messer *et al.* described a bi-allelic polymorphism (NcoI) in the first intron of the TNF-ß gene (TNFB1 and TNFB2) that correlated with a change in the amino acid sequence at position 26.

The single base pair polymorphism at position –308 in the TNF gene is associated with an increased incidence of sepsis and with worse outcome after major trauma and severe burns [29] and in medical and surgical ICU patients [30-33]. However contrary to this, in a comparable patient population not injured or stressed in this way, this association was not observed [34]. The lipopolysaccharide-induced TNF-a production has also been investigated in healthy volunteers and it was found higher among TNF2 carriers. It was concluded that the single base pair polymorphism in position –308 of the TNF gene may influence the production of this cytokine (significantly higher levels of TNF-a were found in the *ex vivo* stimulated blood of heterozygous individuals) [35,36]. Community-acquired pneumonia with subsequent sepsis revealed the same association [37,38]. In Gong's study, the -308A allele was associated with increased 60-day mortality in adult respiratory distress syndrome. However, there was no association between the TNFB polymorphism and adult respiratory distress syndrome mortality [39].

Homozygosity for the TNFB2 allele is associated with an increased incidence of severe sepsis (5.2 times more) and worse outcome [40-42]. Stüber *et al.* examined this polymorphism in septic post-operative patients and found that non-survivors exhibited a significantly higher prevalence of the TNFB2 allele. Homozygous patients for this allele had a higher mortality rate, higher circulating TNF-a concentrations and greater organ dysfunction than heterozygous patients [42,43]. Similar results have been obtained on a medical ICU after severe sepsis [44]. Interestingly, one investigation showed that the observed TNFB2 associations were only present in male septic patients. Female patients displayed normally distributed genotypes without adverse outcomes after sepsis [45]. This polymorphism does not seem to play a role in neonates [46]. However, the neonatal population studied in this investigation was too small for robust statistical analysis.

In severe sepsis, TNF-b NcoI polymorphism is associated with increased mortality. While the genotype TNF-b1/b2 has a higher risk for developing complications, in general the TNF-b2/b2 genotype is associated with more severe complications and mortality from sepsis [47]. However, the influence of polymorphisms of the TNF locus on susceptibility to, and outcome from sepsis is not universally accepted [48].

Specific polymorphism of the TNF-a gene (TNF2 = G to A mutation at the -308 position) and TNF-ß gene (LTA+250 or TNF-ß2) may correlate with higher mortality in septic shock. However, the presence of the A allele at these polymorphic sites did not predispose critically ill surgical patients to either infection or septic shock [49]. Also no correlation between the bi-allelic LT-a (+250 G/A) polymorphism (TNF-ß polymorphism at position +250) and the outcome of critically ill patients was found [50].

Interleukin-1ß (IL-1ß)
The human IL-1 precursor gene was sequenced in 1985 [51]. The IL-1ß gene is located in chromosome 2q14-21 [52,53]. Three polymorphisms of the IL-1ß gene are currently known [54]; position 1903 (T→C) in the promotor region, 5810 (G→A) in intron 4, and 5887 (C→T) in exon 5 [54]. They are associated with different restriction fragment length polymorphism for the endonucleases *Alu*I,

*Bso*FI, and *Taq*I respectively [54,55]. The combination of these three polymorphisms gives rise to the highest information content in comparison to any polymorphism alone [54]. The *Taq*I polymorphism is a 'high-secretor' phenotype (associated with increased secretory levels of IL-1ß) [55]. This secretion was tested *in vitro* in monocyte cultures. However, the *Taq*I polymorphism did not seem to influence outcome after sepsis in a population on a post-operative surgical ICU [44].

Interleukin-6 (IL-6)
The gene for IL-6 was sequenced in 1986 (chromosome 7p21) and at that time it was called B-cell stimulatory factor 2 (BSF-2) [56,57]. IL-6 is a key pro-inflammatory cytokine in the systemic inflammatory response syndrome (SIRS). Increased plasma levels of IL-6 were associated with an adverse outcome after trauma, whereas significantly lower IL-6 plasma concentrations were seen in patients surviving post-traumatic complications [58]. Increased plasma levels of IL-6 were also associated with severe sepsis but not with outcome nor complications after blunt multiple trauma [59,60]. Polymorphisms of IL-6 have been reported in both the 3' and 5' flanking regions and exon 5 [57,61,62]. Two polymorphisms in the 5' flanking region influence restriction sites for *Bgl*I and *Sfa*NI [57, 63]. The *Sfa*NI polymorphism is located at position 174. A homozygotic constellation with this polymorphism (C allele at position –174) coincided with significantly decreased IL-6 serum levels during inflammation, lower total and differential white blood cell count and increased insulin sensitivity than with carriers of the G allele [63-65]. Furthermore, stimulation with lipopolysaccharide or IL-1 resulted in only slightly increased IL-6 secretion in homozygotes, in contrast to heterozygotes [62]. However these associations could not be repeated in Heesen's study [66]. Factors such as circulating endotoxin and lipopolysaccharide binding protein concentration, endotoxin neutralizing capacity, monocyte CD14, soluble CD14 and Toll-like receptors can all affect the IL-6 response to endotoxin [66].

Interestingly in Schluter's study, patients suffering from post-operative severe sepsis had an improved survival with the genotype GG [67]. Haplotype-based analysis of the C/C/G, G/G/G, and G/C/C haplotype clades of IL-6 showed they were strongly associated with increased mortality and more organ dysfunction in the systemic inflammatory response syndrome [68]. Hildebrand *et al.* observed a significantly higher incidence of the allele IL-6 -174G and the homozygous IL-6 -174G genotype in patients with the systemic inflammatory response syndrome [69]. Also, the IL-6 174G/C polymorphism was associated with more serious systemic inflammation as judged by scores based on the values of body temperature, heart rate, respiratory rate and white blood cell count [70].

TNF-a and especially IL-1 related polymorphisms appear to strongly influence cytokine production and outcome in the systemic inflammatory response syndrome or sepsis [71]. An association was found between maximum production of IL-6 and IL-1ß-511*C/T promoter polymorphism [71]. Carriers of less frequent alleles in IL-1-related polymorphisms have a predisposition to excessive IL-6 blood levels and to deterioration in septic shock [71].

Polymorphisms TNF-308*A (single nucleotide polymorphism at position -308 site of the TNF (TNF-308*G/A)), IL1RN*2 and IL1RN*3 (two of the tandem repeat polymorphisms identified within the IL-1 receptor antagonist intron 2 (IL1RN*1-5)) are associated with extremely high IL-6 blood levels and poor outcome in critical illness [72].

Interleukin-10 (IL-10)
The IL-10 gene has been mapped to chromosome 1q31-32, and a number of polymorphisms in the promoter region have been characterized [73-76]. Three single nucleotide polymorphisms at -1082(A/G), -819(C/T), -592(C/A) upstream from the transcription start site [73,76] have been described as well as two additional microsatellite (CA)n repeats, termed IL-10G and IL-10R, located at -1151 and -3978 respectively [74,75]. Variable associations between IL-10 polymorphisms and IL-10 production and autoimmune diseases have been reported [77,78]. Recently published data reveal the influence of different single nucleotide polymorphisms of IL-10 promoter during the development of sepsis; however, these reports are somewhat controversial [79,80,81]. Stanilova *et al.* found that the A allele of the -1082 polymorphism in the IL-10 gene promoter was associated with sepsis susceptibility whereas the G allele was associated with higher stimulated interleukin-10 production and increased mortality in severe sepsis [82].

Pro-inflammatory cytokines such as TNFa [83] and IL-6 [84] are important in the initial phase of the systemic inflammatory response syndrome but are counterbalanced by anti-inflammatory cytokines such as tissue growth factor ß or IL-10, which are considered part of the compensatory anti-inflammatory response syndrome (CARS) [85]. IL-10 (suppressing gene expression of pro-inflammatory cytokines) [86,87] is elevated shortly after trauma [88] and is associated with the development of multiple organ dysfunction. It is now well established that IL-10 single nucleotide polymorphisms are completely (-819 to -592) or strongly linked (-1082 to -819 and -592). In the white population, only 3 haplotypes were found: GCC (G at position -1082, C at position -819 and C at -592), ACC and ATA [76]. These haplotypes have been associated with high (GCC), intermediate (ACC) and low (ATA) IL-10 production [89,90]. Highest IL-10 levels were produced in homozygous GCC/GCC haplotypes [89,90]. The -592A allele has a lower transcriptional activity (decreased IL-10 secretion in *in vitro* studies) [76,79,89]. Patients carrying the genotype -597AC had significantly higher overall organ dysfunction scores and patients carrying the genotype -592AC had a 3.3-fold increase in risk of developing multiple organ dysfunction (but this study's sample size was small) [91].

Genotype distribution of the IL-10 -1082 polymorphism differed significantly between patients and controls. Although the allele frequencies and genotype distribution of the IL-10 -1082 polymorphism did not differ between survivors and non-survivors, patients with severe sepsis were more likely to have the IL-10 -1082 allele 1 [81].

Eskdale *et al*. reported that stimulation of human blood cultures with bacterial lipopolysaccharide showed a genetically-determined large inter-individual variation in IL-10 secretion (>70%). They observed that those haplotypes containing the allele IL10.R3 were associated with lower IL-10 secretion than haplotypes containing any other IL10.R allele. The haplotype IL10.R2/IL10.G14 was associated with highest IL-10 secretion overall while haplotype IL-10.R3/IL10.G7 was associated with the lowest IL-10 secretion [92]. Similar results have been obtained for the dinucleotide repeat at –592 bp [79]. IL-10 is the most potent anti-inflammatory cytokine; it down regulates the production of pro-inflammatory cytokines and chemokines, prevents antigen-specific T-cell activation, inhibits T-cell expansion, and potentiates the release of the inflammatory modulator IL-1ra [87, 93-96]. High IL-10 production correlates with the development of meningococcal disease and other community-acquired infections [79,97]. Genomic polymorphisms within the IL-10 gene have been demonstrated as being associated with inter-individual differences in IL-10 production [76,98]. In critically ill patients, including those with sepsis, IL-10 is increased in circulation and the raised plasma levels correlate with severity and mortality in the inflammatory response [87,93-96].

CRITICAL CARE FOCUS 14: UPDATES

Interleukin-18 (IL-18)

Stassen *et al.* extracted DNA from peripheral leucocytes of trauma patients with an injury severity score =16. Two single nucleotide polymorphisms (-607bp and -137bp) were amplified. Each single nucleotide polymorphism had 2 alleles and 3 genotypes [99]. Individually, each single nucleotide polymorphism had no direct correlation between the patient's genotype and development of infection. However, when the -607bp CA genotype was combined with the -137bp GC genotype (CA/GC), only 4 patients (27%) developed sepsis [99]. This suggests that IL-18 genetic promoter polymorphisms determine the development of post-injury sepsis. Further investigations are needed to identify the impact of variation in genotype across a range of genes involved in connected regulatory pathways [99].

Interferon-γ (IFN-γ)

The outcome of patients with trauma does not always correlate with injury severity or pre-morbid health status. Stassen *et al.* evaluated the relationship between polymorphisms in the first intron of the IFN-γ gene and the development of sepsis after trauma (injury severity score ≤16) [100]. The injury severity score, race, age, and gender distribution were similar for both the septic and non-septic groups. Six alleles and 10 genotypes were identified. Patients who were septic had a 62% chance of having a D allele ($p = 0.06$), whereas they had only a 29% chance of having a C allele. Homozygotes for allele D (DD) were the most likely to become septic (65%) [100] and had an increased chance of developing sepsis after traumatic injury compared with other allelic combinations [100].

ii) Receptors

IL-RN

A significant association between IL-1RN* gene polymorphism (producing interleukin-1 receptor antagonist protein (IL-1Ra) in stimulated peripheral blood mononuclear cells) and survival after severe sepsis was found by Arnalich *et al.* [101]. Homozygotes patients for the allele *2 had a 6.5-fold increased risk of death and produced significantly lower levels of IL-1Ra from their mononuclear cells.

Allele interleukin-1RN2 (interleukin-1 receptor antagonist), but not interleukin-1A or interleukin-1B gene polymorphism, is associated with susceptibility to sepsis. Alleles A2, B2, and RN2 might be important high-risk genetic markers for sepsis [102].

Interferon-γ Receptor 1 (IFN-γR1)

Isolated case reports of germ line defects in the cellular receptor of IFN-γ have been described and mutations characterized [103,104]. There were several non-sense mutations in which receptor truncation resulted in absence of expression. Others were miss-sense mutations in which the binding affinity of the receptor for the ligand was reduced. Moreover, response occurs only after administration of high amounts of exogenous IFN-γ. All affected patients experienced debilitating and unremitting mycobacterial infections [104]. On the basis of these reports it would be worth investigating the potential role of the IFN-γ Receptor 1 gene in infection after major trauma. Indeed, a pilot study conducted by Davis *et al.* revealed that the microsatellite polymorphism AA correlated strongly with infection [105].

Toll-like Receptor 4 (TLR4)

The innate immune system provides an immediate response against toxic insults, mediated by phagocytic cells and host-defence molecules, including pattern recognition receptors (PRRs). An important pattern recognition receptor is TLR4, a transmembrane receptor that recognizes a range of ligands (including lipopolysaccharide); it is found in the cell wall of gram-negative bacteria and plays an important role in their recognition (hTLR4 and CD14 are components of the lipopolysaccharide receptor complex) [106]. A single nucleotide polymorphism in the TLR4 gene, consisting of Asp-299→Gly, leads to hyporesponsiveness to an inhaled lipopolysaccharide charge, reduced airway epithelial TLR4 density, reduced inflammatory cytokine response to lipopolysaccharide, worse clinical outcome and a trend towards an increased mortality [107-111].

hTLR4 mutations are associated with an increased incidence of gram-negative infections in critically ill surgical patients [108]. No association between CD14 polymorphism(s) and the incidence of infection or outcome was observed by Agnese *et al.* [108]. TLR4 Asp299Gly allele was found by Lorenz *et al.* exclusively in patients with septic shock [110]. Furthermore, patients with septic shock with the TLR4 Asp299Gly/Thr399Ile alleles had a higher prevalence of gram-negative infections. It is currently not known whether a hyporesponsive signalling pathway is beneficial or detrimental to the host. Activation of TLR4 has been postulated to be responsible for the pathogenesis of systemic inflammatory response syndrome and TNF-a release [112]. According to Barber *et al.* the TLR4 +896 polymorphism has been associated with an increased risk for severe sepsis following burn trauma [29].

Even in the absence of bacteraemia, patients with the systemic inflammatory response syndrome are prone to an overgrowth of gram-negative bacteria in their small bowel and an increase in mucosal permeability (bacterial translocation) [113]. A number of other factors need to be considered when interpreting these results, including linkage disequilibrium with other single nucleotide polymorphisms in TLR4 or nearby genes which could themselves be causal, and gene–gene interaction with polymorphisms of other genes of the innate immune system (e.g. CD14). Child's preliminary results suggest that TLR4 is biologically plausible as a disease modifying gene [111]. If confirmed, association studies of TLR4 and other genes involved in the innate immune response may identify patients at risk of developing more severe systemic inflammation, who may need closer monitoring and may benefit from more aggressive therapy (e.g. recombinant human activated Protein C).

Toll-like Receptor 2 (TLR2)
Single nucleotide polymorphisms of TLR2 are associated with increased prevalence of positive bacterial cultures and sepsis but not with altered prevalence of septic shock or decreased 28-day survival [114]. Furthermore, TLR2 single nucleotide polymorphisms are associated with gram-positive bacterial infections [114].

Nakada *et al.* investigated the TLR4, CD14, TNF-a, TNF-ß and IL-10 gene polymorphisms in 197 Japanese critically ill patients and 214 healthy control subjects. Their study suggested that TNF-a -308G/A and IL-10-592C/A polymorphisms had a larger effect on clinical outcome of septic patients than the TLR4Asp299Gly, Thr399Ile and CD14-159C/T polymorphisms [115].

iii) Binding Proteins
Lipopolysaccharide binding protein (LBP)
Barber *et al.* suggest that common polymorphisms in the gene for lipopolysaccharide binding protein in combination with male gender are associated with an increased risk of sepsis and, furthermore, may be linked to an unfavourable outcome [116]. These data support the important immunomodulatory role of lipopolysaccharide binding protein in gram-negative sepsis. A single nucleotide polymorphism in the lipopolysaccharide binding protein coding region was reported at the 292 position and results in an amino acid substitution at the adjacent 291 position. This polymorphism does not appear to be associated with complicated sepsis after trauma [117].

Mannose-binding lectin (MBL)
Mannose-binding lectin is an important factor in innate immune defense. The presence of mannose-binding lectin variant alleles (gene polymorphisms causing low levels of mannose-binding lectin) are associated with sepsis, severe sepsis, septic shock and increased risk of fatal outcome [118]. Sutherland *et al.* studied the single nucleotide polymorphisms in mannose-binding lectin and found an increased prevalence of positive bacterial cultures and sepsis but not an altered prevalence of septic shock or decreased 28-day survival [114]. Furthermore, mannose-binding lectin was not associated with a particular organism class [114].

Bactericidal Permeability Increasing Protein (BPI)
Bactericidal permeability increasing protein is a lipid transfer protein, functionally related to lipopolysaccharide binding protein, with high affinity for lipopolysaccharide [119,120]. Bactericidal permeability increasing protein is cytotoxic for gram-negative bacteria but inhibits lipopolysaccharide delivery to the CD14 marker on monocytes [121-123]. Hubacek *et al.* examined the bi-allelic polymorphisms associated with bactericidal permeability increasing protein [116]. No differences in the distribution of the bactericidal permeability increasing protein allelic frequencies was found between septic and control patients. However, a significantly higher number of male septic patients had at least one Cys98Gly allele (when separate comparisons of male/female patients and control groups were made) [116].

CD14
A genetic polymorphism has been identified inside the CD14 promoter sequence (C to T transition at base pair -159) [124-127]. Subjects carrying the T allele have been shown to have significantly higher levels of soluble CD14 than do carriers of the C allele [124,127]. Gibot's *et al.* study demonstrated that the -159TT genotype of the CD14 promoter is associated with susceptibility to and outcome of septic shock [128-130]. The TT genotype frequency was significantly higher in the studied septic shock group than in the control population and appeared to be a genetic risk factor for death attributable to septic shock [128]. High soluble CD14 concentrations are strongly associated with an increased risk of death from septic shock [129,130]. Soluble CD14 promotes microbial components binding to endothelial and epithelial cells, whose ensuing activation may be detrimental [131]. Single nucleotide polymorphisms in CD14 are associated with gram-negative bacteria, increased prevalence of positive bacterial cultures and sepsis but not with altered prevalence of septic shock or decreased 28-day survival [114].

After lipopolysaccharide-stimulation *in vitro*, TT homozygous human monocytes synthesized significantly more soluble CD14 and TNF-a and the T allele had higher promoter activity on gene expression than the C allele [127]. Because CD14 maps to chromosome 5 within a region containing other genes encoding growth factors and interleukins (IL-3, IL-4) [132], Gibot could not exclude the possibility that a linkage disequilibrium between the CD14 polymorphism and these other immune response genes on chromosome 5 may affect the monocytic response to lipopolysaccharide [128].

iv) Other inflammation-related proteins
Surfactant protein-B (SPB)
Polymorphism in intron 4 of the surfactant protein-B gene is associated with adult respiratory distress syndrome and with direct pulmonary injury in women, but not in men. Further studies are needed to confirm the association between the variant surfactant protein-B gene, gender, adult respiratory distress syndrome and direct pulmonary injury [133].

Plasminogen activator inhibitor type 1 glycoprotein (PAI-1)
Plasminogen activator inhibitor type 1 is a pivotal player in the pathogenesis of sepsis and inhibits both tissue- and urokinase-type plasminogen activators. In patients with sepsis, the levels of plasminogen activator inhibitor type 1 are positively related to poor outcome, increased severity of disease, and increased levels of various cytokines, acute phase proteins, and coagulation changes. The 4G/5G insertion/deletion promoter polymorphism, which leads to differences in plasminogen activator inhibitor type 1 production, increases the risk of developing severe complications and dying from sepsis caused by meningococcal infection and multiple trauma [134].

Eriksson *et al.* [135] have shown that plasma plasminogen activator inhibitor type 1 activity is significantly higher in control subjects who are homozygous for the 4G allele than in subjects who are homozygous for the 5G allele. Dawson *et al.* [136] have shown that the response to IL-1 in HepG2 cells is different for the 4G and the 5G allele: the production of mRNA after IL-1 stimulation was 6 times higher in the 4G allele than in the 5G allele.

The plasminogen activator inhibitor type 1 4G allele is associated with high concentrations of plasminogen activator inhibitor type 1 in plasma and a poor survival rate after severe trauma [137]. The increase in plasminogen activator inhibitor type 1 will effectively eliminate plasma tissue-type plasminogen activator, and the microvascular fibrin depositions will no longer be dissolved, resulting in multiorgan failure. It is now well established that the actual levels of plasminogen activator inhibitor type 1 correlate closely with the severity of disseminated intravascular coagulation and are also predictive of final outcome [137-141]. In addition, persisting increased levels predict positively for a bad, often fatal, outcome [142].

Coagulation Factor V
Factor V (component of the prothrombinase complex) influences Protein C activation (anticoagulant) by promoting thrombin generation. Three independent single nucleotide polymorphisms of Factor V in different populations have been described: Factor V Cambridge (Arg306Thr), Factor V Hong Kong (Arg306Gly) and Factor V Leiden (Arg506GLN). They all make Factor Va partially resistant to inactivation by the activated Protein C [143]. In children with meningococcal disease, Factor V Leiden was associated with increased incidence of *purpura fulminans* and a non-statistical trend of reduced mortality [144]. Lower mortality in Factor V Leiden mice was reported after endotoxin exposure, as well as increased thrombin generation and Protein C activation [145]. These observations, in association with previous reports [146] led the authors to speculate that thrombin infusion or optimum generation of thrombin may be beneficial in sepsis, through activation of endogenous Protein C [145].

Tissue Factor
Tissue factor is a membrane protein inducible by endotoxin and thought to be a late factor in sepsis-induced coagulation. It has two promoter haplotypes, 1208D (deletion) and 1208 I (insertion) [147]. The 1208I haplotype has been associated with higher plasma levels of tissue factor and higher risk of venous thrombosis [147].

Thrombomodulin
A point mutation impairing thrombomodulin-mediated Protein C activation is associated with increased mortality to endotoxin in mice [148]. Rare thrombomodulin mutations have been described in families with thromboembolic diseases [149].

Vascular Endothelium Growth Factor (VEGF)
Non-cardiogenic pulmonary oedema is a characteristic feature of the acute respiratory distress syndrome. Medford *et al.* support a role for vascular endothelium growth factor (potent vascular permogen and mitogen) in the pathogenesis of adult respiratory distress syndrome [150]. Lower vascular endothelium growth factor plasma levels have been linked to the presence of the T allele in the +936 CT polymorphism. In patients with adult respiratory distress syndrome

but not those 'at risk', CT and TT genotypes were associated with a higher mean APACHE III score [150].

Renin-Angiotensin
Marshall *et al.* suggest a potential role for renin–angiotensin systems in the pathogenesis of adult respiratory distress syndrome and implicate genetic factors (DD genotype frequency) in the development and progression of this syndrome [151]. Activation of a local renin-angiotensin system within the pulmonary circulation and lung parenchyma could influence the pathogenesis of adult respiratory distress syndrome via a number of mechanisms pertinent to the onset and severity of lung injury. The human angiotensin converting enzyme (ACE) gene contains a polymorphism in which the absence (deletion [D]) rather than the presence (insertion [I]) of a 287-base pair fragment is associated with higher plasma and tissue angiotensin converting enzyme activity [152]. The frequency of the DD angiotensin converting enzyme genotype (associated with higher tissue and circulating angiotensin converting enzyme levels) was increased in the adult respiratory distress syndrome group compared to other ICU patients, after coronary artery bypass grafting or in a UK control group [153]. D allele frequency was also increased in the adult respiratory distress syndrome group and was significantly associated with increased mortality [153].

Heat Shock Proteins (HSP)
Heat shock proteins are thought to play a key role in the recognition of bacterial or viral antigens followed by the production of pro-inflammatory and anti-inflammatory cytokines. Heat shock proteins are cytoprotective molecules expressed in response to a variety of stressful stimuli including heat, microbial infections, ischaemia and inflammatory mediators (e.g. cytokines) [154]. Heat shock proteins, of which the HSP70 family are best understood, respond to stressful stimuli by augmenting intracellular HSP70 gene expression and subsequent inhibition of pro-inflammatory cellular functions [155-157] and also by up-regulation of pro-inflammatory cytokines expression (e.g. TNF and IL-6) [158]. HSP70 also appears to be involved in antigen processing and presentation [159]. These key immunoregulatory functions protect lungs from sepsis-induced injury [160] and macrophages from TNF-induced cell death [161]. There are three genes in the HSP70 family, HSPA1A, HSPA1B and HSPA1L, located adjacent to each other in the class III region of the major histocompatibility complex (chromosome 6p21.3) between the complement and TNF genes [162]. The HSP70 locus in this region suggests a possible role in autoimmune and inflammatory diseases. Nucleotide sequence analysis of the two intronless genes, HSPA1A

and HSPA1B, shows that they encode an identical protein [163]. Both genes are expressed at high levels in cells after heat shock, with HSPA1A also expressed constitutively at very low levels [162]. The HSPA1L gene is expressed at low levels both constitutively and following heat shock, specifically in spermatids [164].

Recently a prospective cohort study of patients with community-acquired pneumonia found that carriage of the HSPA1-B1267*A genotype is associated with a significantly greater risk (relative risk 3.5) of developing septic shock [165]. As HSPA1B1267A>G is a silent mutation, it is likely that another polymorphic site is responsible for the changes in biological function that explain the disease association [165]. Genetic variants of the HSP70 genes, in particular the HSPA1B1267A>G, HSPA1A-27G>C, and HSPA1L2437C>T polymorphisms, have been implicated in several inflammatory and autoimmune disease conditions [166]. These studies combined with the finding that the 'functional' polymorphic site is likely to be close to HSPA1B [165], suggest that HSPA1A and HSPA1B are good candidates to search for the 'functional' polymorphic site of the haplotype. Temple *et al.* [167] hypothesized that there are polymorphic sites within HSPA1A and HSPA1B in linkage with HSPA1B1267A>G. Furthermore, they hypothesized that some of these polymorphic sites influence lipopolysaccharide-stimulated production of HSPA1A and HSPA1B by peripheral blood mononuclear cells.

HSPA1B-179C>T was found to be in linkage disequilibrium with HSPA1B1267A>G and is associated with variable production of HSPA1B and HSPA1A production [167]. This suggests that HSPA1B-179C>T affects HSP70 production and is a key determinant of individual susceptibility to a variety of infectious and inflammatory diseases (such as HIV/AIDS, asthma, common bacterial and parasitic infections, inflammatory bowel disease and rheumatoid arthritis) [167].

Apolipoprotein E (APOE)
Although precise mechanisms leading to organ dysfunction in severe sepsis remain incompletely understood, the role of lipid mediators has been suggested [168-171]. Recent evidence suggests that there is a link between lipoproteins and apolipoproteins, general host inflammatory responses [172] and sepsis outcome [171-174]. Apolipoprotein E-deficient animals display impaired immune responses and increased susceptibility to endotoxemia and bacterial and fungal infections [175-177]. Exogenous administration of apolipoprotein E or apolipoprotein E-mimetic peptides in animals

suppresses local as well as systematic inflammatory responses [178] and decreases mortality [179]. Independent of lipoprotein transport, apolipoprotein E can have a dual pro- or anti- inflammatory effect [180,181]. This dual effect could be explained by cell-specific differences in apolipoprotein E isoform binding [182,183].

In an elective surgical cohort studied by Moretti *et al.*, the presence of the apolipoprotein e3 allelic variant of the apolipoprotein E gene was associated with decreased incidence of severe sepsis and a shorter ICU length of stay [184]. Apolipoprotein E genotypes were not associated with parameters such as duration of mechanical ventilation or ICU mortality [184].

Migration Inhibitory Factor (MIF)
Migration inhibitory factor is a pro-inflammatory cytokine having a wide variety of functions [185-187]. Mice treated with anti-migration inhibitory factor antibodies were protected from lipopolysaccharide-induced lethality [188,189]. Elevated migration inhibitory factor plasma levels are associated with poor outcomes in septic patients [190-192]. Polymorphisms in the promoter region of the migration inhibitory factor gene have been identified (-173G→C and -794 VNTR of 5 to 8 repeats) [193-195]. The -173G→C polymorphism has been associated to various inflammatory diseases such as juvenile idiopathic arthritis [10,193-195].

Discussion
During the past decade, with the availability of improved molecular diagnostic techniques, 'disease-gene association' studies have investigated the role of genetic variations in the inflammatory response to infection. Specific treatment strategies with biological response modifiers have entered phase II clinical trials but so far without success. Possible reasons could be the difficulty in identifying the patients who might benefit from this type of therapy and the critical delay between the onset of complications (e.g. sepsis, adult respiratory distress syndrome, multiple organ dysfunction) and the treatment. This may be overcome by the latest techniques in molecular biology and genetics by quickly identifying high-risk patients. A growing body of evidence now suggests that genetic susceptibility influences the development of surgical sepsis and adult respiratory distress syndrome and multiple organ dysfunction. Functional polymorphisms in several cytokine genes provide a potential mechanism whereby these variations may be identified.

Sepsis is a polygenic syndrome and allelic variants in multiple genes have an impact on the clinical outcome. It is unlikely that one polymorphism will result in a particular phenotype but when several polymorphisms act together in the presence of infection, the disease phenotype associated with a defined outcome may be apparent. The majority of single nucleotide polymorphisms have no impact on biological function. The inflammatory response operates both in series and in parallel, in a highly complex network, with a substantial degree of redundancy. Hence, even a single functional polymorphism is unlikely to influence the overall inflammatory response in more than a fraction of the patients [196]. Large groups of patients are required to demonstrate a significant, yet rather small, association between a single nucleotide polymorphism and a clinical event [196]. When single nucleotide polymorphism assessments are employed as a tool to predict the clinical course of ICU patients, a large number of single nucleotide polymorphisms should ideally be examined simultaneously. This method would identify unfortunate combinations of single nucleotide polymorphisms and would have higher predictive power [196].

When investigating genetic polymorphisms, it is not enough just to determine the presence of a polymorphism. One has to take several criteria into account. Patients do show different genetic constitutions. Investigating polymorphisms linked to disease can be blurred by existing genetic variation. Therefore, it is necessary to determine the overall genetic constellation of the population under investigation. Furthermore, the power of the study has to be sufficient to explore a specific hypothesis. One has to consider whether other genes may be involved. Such genes might be the actual cause for any differences detected. The investigated gene may then just be an epiphenomenon. It is therefore important to study family genetics at the same time. The family constitution can reveal more about underlying genes involved in the disease process. If differences in disease outcome are linked to one or more genetic polymorphisms, one has to perform a subsequent study in another cohort. This cohort has to show similar linkage of genes to outcome. Thus, investigating genetic polymorphisms should adhere to some basic rules listed in Table 2.

Table 2. Validation criteria for studying genetic polymorphisms.

Overall genetic constellation of the population
Power of the study
Other genetic associations/epiphenomena
Family genetics
Reproducibility in a second cohort
Prospective or retrospective study

CRITICAL CARE FOCUS 14: UPDATES

Currently, a number of studies suggest that specific polymorphic variants are important determining the severity and outcome from post-traumatic sepsis. However, not all of the above reported studies fulfill the criteria mentioned. Despite the available evidence, larger scale studies adhering to specific genetic association criteria are needed.

Future research should focus on a broad array of genes. Single nucleotide polymorphisms genotyping assays (micro-array techniques) can achieve this and so categorize patients. Early identification of patients at risk would direct interventions which modify the biological response to improve morbidity and mortality rates. Early-goal directed therapy, low-dose steroid supplementation, blood glucose control and activated Protein C therapy appear to be associated with an improved outcome after sepsis [197-202].

Further advances will improve understanding of how genetic variability influences responses to infection and pharmacotherapy. In the near future, genetic information obtained at disease presentation will help to predict outcome and will enable selection of a 'genetic' drug.

It is important to keep in mind however, that most of the published studies have small sample size, with geographic and not necessarily ethnic distinction. Because of the limited groups examined and the fact that not all studies have adhered to specific genetic association criteria, application of genetic information to patients will need multicentre and multinational studies.

Glossary

Allele: Alternative form of a genetic locus; a single allele for each locus is inherited separately from each parent (e.g. at a locus for eye colour the allele might result in blue or brown eyes). Thus an allele is any of two or more alternative forms of a gene that occupy the same locus on a chromosome.

Codon: The coding unit of DNA that specifies the function of the corresponding messenger RNA.

Endonuclease restriction sites: An endonuclease (enzyme) that binds to double-stranded DNA at a specific nucleotide sequence (site) and then, if both strands of the DNA lack appropriate modification at that sequence, cleaves the DNA either at the recognition sequence or at another site in the DNA molecule.

Exon: The protein-coding DNA sequence of a gene. A segment of a gene that contains instructions for making a protein. In many genes the exons are separated by 'intervening' segments of DNA, known as introns, which do not code for proteins; these introns are removed by splicing to produce messenger RNA.

Flanking region: The DNA sequences extending on either side of a specific locus or gene. For microsatellites, the flanking regions are the stretches of DNA outside the simple sequence tandem repeat (STR). These sequences are used as primer pairs. The flanking regions are usually invariant across a population or species, but mutations in the flanking region can be a cause of null alleles as well as a potentially serious source of homoplasy.

Haplotype: Set of allelic states found at neighbouring loci in a chromosome, as inherited from a parent. Haplotypes can be broken down by recombination. A haplotype shared among unrelated individuals affected with a genetic disease may indicate that a gene causing the disease maps to that genomic region. Thus haptotypes are a set of closely linked alleles (genes or DNA polymorphisms) inherited as a unit. Different combinations of polymorphisms are known as haplotypes. Collectively the results from several loci could be referred to as a haplotype. 'Haplo' comes from the Greek word for 'single'.

Haplotype Clades: Multiple haplotypes exist for all studied genes; thus, grouping haplotypes into haplotype clades (evolutionarily related groups of haplotypes) increases the statistical power to associate genotype with phenotype.

Intron: The DNA base sequence interrupting the protein coding sequence of a gene; this sequence is transcribed into RNA but is cut out of the message before it is translated into protein. An intron is a region of DNA that does not code for the synthesis of a protein or a section of a gene that does not contain any instructions for making a protein. Introns separate exons - the coding sections - from each other.

Intronless genes: Eukaryotic genes are either 'intron containing' or 'intronless'.

Linkage disequilibrium: Linkage disequilibrium is often termed 'allelic association.' When alleles at two distinctive loci occur in gametes more frequently than expected given the known allele frequencies and recombination fraction between the two loci, the alleles are said to be in linkage disequilibrium. Evidence for linkage disequilibrium can be helpful in mapping disease genes since it suggests that the two may be very close to one another.

Microsatellite repeat: Microsatellites are defined as loci (or regions within DNA sequences) where short sequences of DNA (nucleotides; adenine - A, thiamine - T, guanine - G, cytosine - C) are repeated in tandem arrays. This means that the sequences are repeated one right after the other. The lengths of sequences used most often are di-, tri-, or tetra-nucleotides. What makes microsatellites useful is the fact that at the same location within the genomic DNA the number of times the sequence (e.g. AC) is repeated often varies between individuals, within populations, and/or between species. So one population may commonly have 13 ACs repeated in a row while another population has 18 ACs repeated at the same location within the genomic DNA. Different regions of the DNA contain sequences that mutate at various rates. Some regions have a high rate of mutation while others have a low rate of change. In areas of the genome with high rates of mutation there is a wider range in the number of repeats found within individuals of a population (some individuals have 10 repeats others 11, 13, or more repeats). Each sequence with a specific number of repeated nucleotides is designated as an *allele*. So, a *locus* (a specific region within the genomic DNA) with 8 repeats is one allele and within another individual the same locus that contains 9 repeats is another allele.

Mis-sense mutations: A mutation that changes a codon for one amino acid into a codon specifying another amino acid. A mutation that alters a codon for a particular amino acid to one specifying a different amino acid.

Mitogen: a substance that induces cell division.

Non-sense mutation: A single base pair substitution that prematurely codes for a stop in amino acid translation (stop codon).

Permogen: Agent/molecule having the capability to induce/increase the vascular permeability. Vascular endothelium growth factor has been identified as a key molecule in the control of vascular permeability via interactions with the endothelial cell.

Polymorphism: A naturally occurring variation in the sequence of genetic information on a segment of DNA among individuals.

Promoter: DNA sequence that enables a gene to be transcribed. The promoter is recognized by RNA polymerase, which then initiates transcription. In RNA synthesis, promoters are a means to demarcate which genes should be used for messenger RNA creation and, by extension, control which proteins the cell manufactures.

Restriction fragment: the fragment of DNA that is produced by cleaving DNA with a restriction enzyme.

Restriction site: A specific nucleotide sequence in duplex DNA recognized and cleaved by a restriction endonuclease.

Surface receptor: Cell surface receptors are integral membrane proteins and, as such, have regions that contribute to three basic domains:
Extracellular domains: Some of the residues exposed to the outside of the cell interact with and bind the hormone - another term for these regions is the *ligand-binding domain*.
Transmembrane domains: Hydrophobic stretches of amino acids are 'comfortable' in the lipid bilayer and serve to anchor the receptor in the membrane.
Cytoplasmic or intracellular domains: Tails or loops of the receptor that are within the cytoplasm react to hormone binding by interacting in some way with other molecules, leading to generation of second messengers. Cytoplasmic residues of the receptor are thus the *effector region* of the molecule.
Several distinctive variations in receptor structure have been identified. Some receptors are simple, single-pass proteins; many growth factor receptors take this form. Others, such as the receptor for insulin, have more than one subunit. Another class, which includes the beta-adrenergic receptor, is threaded through the membrane seven times.

Transcription Start Site: Transcription is the process whereby RNA copies are made from sections of the DNA genome. Transcription is directed by promoter regions. These define the transcription start site, and also the set of cellular conditions under which the promoter is active. At least in more complex species, it appears to be common for genes to have several different transcription start sites, which may be active under different conditions.

References
1. Nast-Kolb D, Waydhas C, Gippner-Steppert C, *et al*. Indicators of the posttraumatic inflammatory response correlate with organ

failure in patients with multiple injuries. Journal of Trauma 1997; 42; 446-454.
2. Tompkins RG. The role of proinflammatory cytokines in inflammatory and metabolic responses. Annals of Surgery 1997; 225: 243-245.
3. Cipolle MD, Pasquale MD, Cerra FB. Secondary organ dysfunction. From clinical perspectives to molecular mediators. Critical Care Clinics 1993; 9: 261-298.
4. Polk HC, Jr. Non-specific host defence stimulation in the reduction of surgical infection in man. British Journal of Surgery 1987; 74: 969-970.
5. Abraham E. Host defense abnormalities after hemorrhage, trauma, and burns. Critical Care Medicine 1989; 17: 934-939.
6. Smith RM, Giannoudis PV. Trauma and the immune response. Journal of the Royal Society of Medicine 1998; 91: 417-420.
7. Giannoudis PV, Smith RM, Banks RE, Windsor AC, Dickson RA, Guillou PJ. Stimulation of inflammatory markers after blunt trauma. British Journal of Surgery 1998; 85: 986-990.
8. Hoch RC, Rodriguez R, Manning T, *et al*. Effects of accidental trauma on cytokine and endotoxin production. Critical Care Medicine 1993; 21: 839-845.
9. Guillou PJ. Biological variation in the development of sepsis after surgery or trauma. Lancet 1993; 342: 217-220.
10. Amoli MM, Shelley E, Mattey DL, *et al.* Intercellular adhesion molecule-1 gene polymorphisms in isolated polymyalgia rheumatica. Journal of Rheumatology 2002; 29: 502-504.
11. Buxbaum JD, Silverman JM, Smith CJ, *et al*. Association between a GABRB3 polymorphism and autism. Molecular Psychiatry 2002; 7: 311-316.
12. Cuthbert AP, Fisher SA, Mirza MM, *et al*. The contribution of NOD2 gene mutations to the risk and site of disease in inflammatory bowel disease. Gastroenterology 2002; 122: 867-874.
13. Forton AC, Petri MA, Goldman D, Sullivan KE. An osteopontin (SPP1) polymorphism is associated with systemic lupus erythematosus. Human Mutation 2002; 19: 459.
14. Hyndman ME, Parsons HG, Verma S, *et al*. The T-786-->C mutation in endothelial nitric oxide synthase is associated with hypertension. Hypertension 2002; 39: 919-922.
15. Kojima Y, Kinouchi Y, Takahashi S, Negoro K, Hiwatashi N, Shimosegawa T. Inflammatory bowel disease is associated with a novel promoter polymorphism of natural resistance-associated macrophage protein 1 (NRAMP1) gene. Tissue Antigens 2001; 58: 379-384.

16. Niu T, Chen X, Xu X. Angiotensin converting enzyme gene insertion/deletion polymorphism and cardiovascular disease: therapeutic implications. Drugs 2002; 62: 977-993.
17. Rayner ML, Kelly MA, Cordell HJ, McTernan CL, Mijovic CH, Barnett AH. Analysis of the role of DPB1-encoded amino acids in the genetic predisposition to type I diabetes mellitus. Human Immunology 2002; 6: 413-417.
18. Sakurai K, Migita O, Toru M, Arinami T. An association between a missense polymorphism in the close homologue of L1 (CHL1, CALL) gene and schizophrenia. Molecular Psychiatry 2002; 7: 412-415.
19. Wang XL, Greco M, Sim AS, Duarte N, Wang J, Wilcken DE. Effect of CYP1A1 MspI polymorphism on cigarette smoking related coronary artery disease and diabetes. Atherosclerosis 2002; 16: 391-397.
20. Chen HY, Chen WC, Hsu CD, Tsai FJ, Tsai CH. Relation of vitamin D receptor FokI start codon polymorphism to bone mineral density and occurrence of osteoporosis in postmenopausal women in Taiwan. Acta Obstetricia et Gynecologica Scandinavica 2002; 8: 93-98.
21. Nishijima S, Sugaya K, Naito A, Morozumi M, Hatano T, Ogawa Y. Association of vitamin D receptor gene polymorphism with urolithiasis. Journal of Urology 2002; 167: 2188-2191.
22. Xu PY, Liang R, Jankovic J, Hunter C, *et al*. Association of homozygous 7048G7049 variant in the intron six of Nurr1 gene with Parkinson's disease. Neurology 2002; 58: 881-884.
23. Rossetti S, Burton S, Strmecki L, *et al*. The position of the polycystic kidney disease 1 (PKD1) gene mutation correlates with the severity of renal disease. Journal of the American Society of Nephrology 2002; 13: 1230-1237.
24. Wang X, DeKosky ST, Luedecking-Zimmer E, Ganguli M, Kamboh IM. Genetic variation in alpha (1)-antichymotrypsin and its association with Alzheimer's disease. Human Genetics 2002; 110: 356-365.
25. Nedospasov SA, Shakhov AN, Turetskaya RL, *et al*. Tandem arrangement of genes coding for tumor necrosis factor (TNF-alpha) and lymphotoxin (TNF-beta) in the human genome. Cold Spring Harbor Symposia on Quantitative Biology 1986; 51: 611-624.
26. Beutler B, Cerami A. The biology of cachectin/TNF--a primary mediator of the host response. Annual Review of Immunology 1989; 7: 625-655.
27. Wilson AG, de VN, Pociot F, di Giovine FS, van der Putte LB, Duff GW. An allelic polymorphism within the human tumor

necrosis factor alpha promoter region is strongly associated with HLA A1, B8, and DR3 alleles. Journal of Experimental Medicine 1993; 177: 557-560.
28. Messer G, Spengler U, Jung MC, *et al.* Polymorphic structure of the tumor necrosis factor (TNF) locus: an NcoI polymorphism in the first intron of the human TNF-beta gene correlates with a variant amino acid in position 26 and a reduced level of TNF-beta production. Journal of Experimental Medicine 1991; 173: 209-219.
29. Barber RC, Aragaki CC, Rivera-Chavez FA, Purdue GF, Hunt JL, Horton JW. TLR4 and TNF-alpha polymorphisms are associated with an increased risk for severe sepsis following burn injury. Journal of Medical Genetics 2004; 41: 808-813.
30. Majetschak M, Obertacke U, Schade FU, *et al.* Tumor necrosis factor gene polymorphisms, leukocyte function, and sepsis susceptibility in blunt trauma patients. Clinical and Diagnostic Laboratory Immunology 2002; 9: 1205-1211.
31. O'Keefe GE, Hybki DL, Munford RS. The G-->A single nucleotide polymorphism at the -308 position in the tumor necrosis factor-alpha promoter increases the risk for severe sepsis after trauma. Journal of Trauma 2002; 52: 817-825.
32. Tang GJ, Huang SL, Yien HW, *et al.* Tumor necrosis factor gene polymorphism and septic shock in surgical infection. Critical Care Medicine 2000; 28: 2733-2736.
33. Mira JP, Cariou A, Grall F, *et al.* Association of TNF2, a TNF-alpha promoter polymorphism, with septic shock susceptibility and mortality: a multicenter study. Journal of the American Medical Association 1999; 282: 561-568.
34. Stuber F, Udalova IA, Book M, *et al.* -308 tumor necrosis factor (TNF) polymorphism is not associated with survival in severe sepsis and is unrelated to lipopolysaccharide inducibility of the human TNF promoter. Journal of Inflammation 1995; 46: 42-50.
35. Heesen M, Kunz D, Bachmann-Mennenga B, Merk HF, Bloemeke B. Linkage disequilibrium between tumor necrosis factor (TNF)-alpha-308 G/A promoter and TNF-beta NcoI polymorphisms: Association with TNF-alpha response of granulocytes to endotoxin stimulation. Critical Care Medicine 2003; 31: 211-214.
36. Louis E, Franchimont D, Piron A, *et al.* Tumour necrosis factor (TNF) gene polymorphism influences TNF-alpha production in lipopolysaccharide (LPS)-stimulated whole blood cell culture in healthy humans. Clinical and Experimental Immunology 1998; 113: 401-406.
37. Waterer GW, Wunderink RG. Genetic susceptibility to pneumonia. Clinics in Chest Medicine 2005; 2: 29-38.

38. Wunderink RG, Waterer GW, Cantor RM, and Quasney MW. Tumor necrosis factor gene polymorphisms and the variable presentation and outcome of community-acquired pneumonia. Chest 2002; 121: 87S-88S.
39. Gong MN, Zhou W, Williams PL, *et al.* 308GA and TNFB polymorphisms in acute respiratory distress syndrome. European Respiratory Journal 2005; 26: 382-389.
40. Flach R, Majetschak M, Heukamp T, *et al.* Relation of ex vivo stimulated blood cytokine synthesis to post-traumatic sepsis. Cytokine 1999; 11; 173-178.
41. Majetschak M, Flohe S, Obertacke U, *et al.* Relation of a TNF gene polymorphism to severe sepsis in trauma patients. Annals of Surgery 1999; 230: 207-214.
42. Reid CL, Perrey C, Pravica V, Hutchinson IV, Campbell IT. Genetic variation in proinflammatory and anti-inflammatory cytokine production in multiple organ dysfunction syndrome. Critical Care Medicine 2002; 30: 2216-2221.
43. Stuber F, Petersen M, Bokelmann F, Schade U. A genomic polymorphism within the tumor necrosis factor locus influences plasma tumor necrosis factor-alpha concentrations and outcome of patients with severe sepsis. Critical Care Medicine 1996; 24: 381-384.
44. Fang XM, Schroder S, Hoeft A, Stuber F. Comparison of two polymorphisms of the interleukin-1 gene family: interleukin-1 receptor antagonist polymorphism contributes to susceptibility to severe sepsis. Critical Care Medicine 1999; 27: 1330-1334.
45. Schroder J, Kahlke V, Book M, Stuber F. Gender differences in sepsis: genetically determined? Shock 2000; 14: 307-310.
46. Weitkamp JH, Stuber F, Bartmann P. Pilot study assessing TNF gene polymorphism as a prognostic marker for disease progression in neonates with sepsis. Infection 2000; 28: 92-96.
47. Kahlke V, Schafmayer C, Schniewind B, Seegert D, Schreiber S, Schroder J. Are postoperative complications genetically determined by TNF-beta NcoI gene polymorphism? Surgery 2004; 135: 365-373.
48. Gordon AC, Lagan AL, Aganna E, *et al.* TNF and TNFR polymorphisms in severe sepsis and septic shock: a prospective multicentre study. Genes and Immunity 2004; 5: 631-640.
49. Calvano JE, Um JY, Agnese DM, *et al.* Influence of the TNF-alpha and TNF-beta polymorphisms upon infectious risk and outcome in surgical intensive care patients. Surgical Infections (Larchmt) 2003; 4: 163-169.
50. Rauchschwalbe SK, Maseizik T, Mittelkotter U, *et al.* Effect of the LT-alpha (+250 G/A) polymorphism on markers of

inflammation and clinical outcome in critically ill patients. Journal of Trauma 2004; 56: 815-822.
51. Furutani Y, Notake M, Yamayoshi M, *et al*. Cloning and characterization of the cDNAs for human and rabbit interleukin-1 precursor. Nucleic Acids Research 1985; 13: 5869-5882.
52. Steinkasserer A, Spurr NK, Cox S, Jeggo P, Sim RB. The human IL-1 receptor antagonist gene (IL1RN) maps to chromosome 2q14-q21, in the region of the IL-1 alpha and IL-1 beta loci. Genomics 1992; 13: 654-657.
53. Webb AC, Collins KL, Auron PE, *et al*. Interleukin-1 gene (IL1) assigned to long arm of human chromosome 2. Lymphokine Research, 1986; 5: 77-85.
54. Guasch JF, Bertina RM, Reitsma PH. Five novel intragenic dimorphisms in the human interleukin-1 genes combine to high informativity. Cytokine 1996; 8: 598-602.
55. Pociot F, Molvig J, Wogensen L, Worsaae H, Nerup J. A TaqI polymorphism in the human interleukin-1 beta (IL-1 beta) gene correlates with IL-1 beta secretion in vitro. European Journal of Clinical Investigation 1992; 22: 396-402.
56. Hirano T, Yasukawa K, Harada H, *et al*. Complementary DNA for a novel human interleukin (BSF-2) that induces B lymphocytes to produce immunoglobulin. Nature 1986; 324: 73-76.
57. Bowcock AM, Kidd JR, Lathrop GM, *et al*. The human "interferon-beta 2/hepatocyte stimulating factor/interleukin-6" gene: DNA polymorphism studies and localization to chromosome 7p21. Genomics 1988; 3: 8-16.
58. Seekamp A, Jochum M, Ziegler M, van GM, Martin M, Regel G. Cytokines and adhesion molecules in elective and accidental trauma-related ischemia/reperfusion. Journal of Trauma 1998; 44: 874-882.
59. Doughty LA, Kaplan SS, Carcillo JA. Inflammatory cytokine and nitric oxide responses in pediatric sepsis and organ failure. Critical Care Medicine 1996; 24: 1137-1143.
60. Giannoudis PV, Smith MR, Evans RT, Bellamy MC, Guillou PJ. Serum CRP and IL-6 levels after trauma. Not predictive of septic complications in 31 patients. Acta Orthopaedica Scandinavica 1998; 69: 184-188.
61. Bowcock AM, Ray A, Erlich H, Sehgal PB. Rapid detection and sequencing of alleles in the 3' flanking region of the interleukin-6 gene. Nucleic Acids Research 1989; 17: 6855-6864.
62. Fishman D, Faulds G, Jeffery R, *et al*. The effect of novel polymorphisms in the interleukin-6 (IL-6) gene on IL-6 transcription and plasma IL-6 levels, and an association with

systemic-onset juvenile chronic arthritis. Journal of Clinical Investigation 1998; 102: 1369-1376.

63. Osiri M, McNicholl J, Moreland LW, Bridges SL, Jr. A novel single nucleotide polymorphism and five probable haplotypes in the 5' flanking region of the IL-6 gene in African-Americans. Genes and Immunity 1999; 1: 166-167.

64. Fernandez-Real JM, Broch M, Vendrell J, et al. Interleukin-6 gene polymorphism and insulin sensitivity. Diabetes 2000; 49: 517-520.

65. Montgomery HE, Marshall R, Hemingway H, et al. Human gene for physical performance. Nature 1998; 393: 221-222.

66. Heesen M, Obertacke U, Schade FU, Bloemeke B, Majetschak M. The interleukin-6 G(-174)C polymorphism and the ex vivo interleukin-6 response to endotoxin in severely injured blunt trauma patients. European Cytokine Network 2002; 13: 72-77.

67. Schluter B, Raufhake C, Erren M, et al. Effect of the interleukin-6 promoter polymorphism (-174 G/C) on the incidence and outcome of sepsis. Critical Care Medicine 2002; 30: 32-37.

68. Sutherland AM, Walley KR, Manocha S, Russell JA. The association of interleukin 6 haplotype clades with mortality in critically ill adults. Archives of Internal Medicine 2005; 165: 75-82.

69. Hildebrand F, Pape HC, Griensven M, et al. Genetic predisposition for a compromised immune system after multiple trauma. Shock 2005; 24; 518-522.

70. American College of Chest Physicians/Society of Critical Care Medicine Consensus Conference. Definitions for sepsis and organ failure and guidelines for the use of innovative therapies in sepsis. Critical Care Medicine 1992; 20: 864-874.

71. Watanabe E, Hirasawa H, Oda S, et al. Cytokine-related genotypic differences in peak interleukin-6 blood levels of patients with SIRS and septic complications. Journal of Trauma 2005; 59: 1181-1189.

72. Watanabe E, Hirasawa H, Oda S, Matsuda K, Hatano M, Tokuhisa T. Extremely high interleukin-6 blood levels and outcome in the critically ill are associated with tumor necrosis factor- and interleukin-1-related gene polymorphisms. Critical Care Medicine 2005; 33: 89-97.

73. D'Alfonso S, Rampi M, Rolando V, Giordano M, Momigliano-Richiardi P. New polymorphisms in the IL-10 promoter region. Genes and Immunity 2000; 1: 231-233.

74. Eskdale J, Gallagher G. A polymorphic dinucleotide repeat in the human IL-10 promoter. Immunogenetics 1995; 42: 444-445.

75. Eskdale J, Kube D, Tesch H, Gallagher G. Mapping of the human IL10 gene and further characterization of the 5' flanking sequence. Immunogenetics 1997; 46: 120-128.
76. Turner DM, Williams DM, Sankaran D, Lazarus M, Sinnott PJ, Hutchinson IV. An investigation of polymorphism in the interleukin-10 gene promoter. Europeasn Journal of Immunogenetics 1997; 24: 1-8.
77. D'Alfonso S, Rampi M, Bocchio D, Colombo G, Scorza-Smeraldi R, Momigliano-Richardi P. Systemic lupus erythematosus candidate genes in the Italian population: evidence for a significant association with interleukin-10. Arthritis and Rheumatism 2000; 43: 120-128.
78. Eskdale J, McNicholl J, Wordsworth P, et al. Interleukin-10 microsatellite polymorphisms and IL-10 locus alleles in rheumatoid arthritis susceptibility. Lancet 1998; 352: 1282-1283.
79. Lowe PR, Galley HF, bdel-Fattah A, Webster NR. Influence of interleukin-10 polymorphisms on interleukin-10 expression and survival in critically ill patients. Critical Care Medicine 2003; 31: 34-38.
80. Schaaf BM, Boehmke F, Esnaashari H, et al. Pneumococcal septic shock is associated with the interleukin-10-1082 gene promoter polymorphism. American Journal of Respiratory and Critical Care Medicine 2003; 168: 476-480.
81. Shu Q, Fang X, Chen Q, Stuber F. IL-10 polymorphism is associated with increased incidence of severe sepsis. Chinese Medical Journal (Engl) 2003;116: 1756-1759.
82. Stanilova SA, Miteva LD, Karakolev ZT, Stefanov CS. Interleukin-10-1082 promoter polymorphism in association with cytokine production and sepsis susceptibility. Intensive Care Medicine 2006; 32: 260-266.
83. Pellegrini JD, Puyana JC, Lapchak PH, Kodys K, Miller-Graziano CL. A membrane TNF-alpha/TNFR ratio correlates to MODS score and mortality. Shock 1996; 6: 389-396.
84. Gebhard F, Pfetsch H, Steinbach G, Strecker W, Kinzl L, Bruckner UB. Is interleukin 6 an early marker of injury severity following major trauma in humans? Archives of Surgery 2000; 135: 291-295.
85. Molloy RG, Mannick JA, Rodrick ML. Cytokines, sepsis and immunomodulation. British Journal of Surgery 1993; 80: 289-297.
86. Moore KW, de Waal MR, Coffman RL, O'Garra A. Interleukin-10 and the interleukin-10 receptor. Annual Review of Immunology 2001; 19: 683-765.

87. Oberholzer A, Oberholzer C, Moldawer LL. Interleukin-10: A complex role in the pathogenesis of sepsis syndromes and its potential as an anti-inflammatory drug. Critical Care Medicine 2002; 30: S58-S63.
88. Neidhardt R, Keel M, Steckholzer U, *et al*. Relationship of interleukin-10 plasma levels to severity of injury and clinical outcome in injured patients. Journal of Trauma 1997; 42: 863-870.
89. Crawley E, Kay R, Sillibourne J, Patel P, Hutchinson I, Woo P. Polymorphic haplotypes of the interleukin-10 5' flanking region determine variable interleukin-10 transcription and are associated with particular phenotypes of juvenile rheumatoid arthritis. Arthritis and Rheumatism 1999; 42: 1101-1108.
90. Edwards-Smith CJ, Jonsson JR, Purdie DM, Bansal A, Shorthouse C, Powell EE. Interleukin-10 promoter polymorphism predicts initial response of chronic hepatitis C to interferon alfa. Hepatology 1999; 30: 526-530.
91. Schroder O, Laun RA, Held B, Ekkernkamp A, Schulte KM. Association of interleukin-10 promoter polymorphism with the incidence of multiple organ dysfunction following major trauma: results of a prospective pilot study. Shock 2004; 21: 306-310.
92. Eskdale J, Gallagher G, Verweij CL, Keijsers V, Westendorp RG, Huizinga TW. Interleukin 10 secretion in relation to human IL-10 locus haplotypes. Procedings of the National Academy of Science of the USA 1998; 95: 9465-9470.
93. Kahlke V, Dohm C, Mees T, Brotzmann K, Schreiber S, Schroder J. Early interleukin-10 treatment improves survival and enhances immune function only in males after hemorrhage and subsequent sepsis. Shock 2002; 18: 24-28.
94. Latifi SQ, O'Riordan MA, Levine AD. Interleukin-10 controls the onset of irreversible septic shock. Infection and Immunity 2002; 70: 4441-4446.
95. Loisa P, Rinne T, Laine S, Hurme M, Kaukinen S. Anti-inflammatory cytokine response and the development of multiple organ failure in severe sepsis. Acta Anaesthesiologica Scandinavica 2003; 47: 319-325.
96. Lyons A, Kelly JL, Rodrick ML, Mannick JA, Lederer JA. Major injury induces increased production of interleukin-10 by cells of the immune system with a negative impact on resistance to infection. Annals of Surgery 1997; 226: 450-458.
97. Westendorp RG, Langermans JA, Huizinga TW, *et al*. Genetic influence on cytokine production and fatal meningococcal disease. Lancet 1997; 349: 170-173.

98. Gallagher PM, Lowe G, Fitzgerald T, et al. Association of IL-10 polymorphism with severity of illness in community acquired pneumonia. Thorax 2003; 58: 154-156.
99. Stassen NA, Breit CM, Norfleet LA, Polk HC, Jr. IL-18 promoter polymorphisms correlate with the development of post-injury sepsis. Surgery 2003; 134: 351-356.
100. Stassen NA, Leslie-Norfleet LA, Robertson AM, Eichenberger MR, Polk HC, Jr. Interferon-gamma gene polymorphisms and the development of sepsis in patients with trauma. Surgery 2002; 132: 289-292.
101. Arnalich F, Lopez-Maderuelo D, Codoceo R, et al. Interleukin-1 receptor antagonist gene polymorphism and mortality in patients with severe sepsis. Clinical and Experimental Immunology 2002; 127: 331-336.
102. Ma P, Chen D, Pan J, Du B. Genomic polymorphism within interleukin-1 family cytokines influences the outcome of septic patients. Critical Care Medicine 2002; 30: 1046-1050.
103. Jouanguy E, Altare F, Lamhamedi S, et al. Interferon-gamma-receptor deficiency in an infant with fatal bacille Calmette-Guerin infection. New England Journal of Medicine 1996; 335: 1956-1961.
104. Newport MJ, Huxley CM, Huston S, et al. A mutation in the interferon-gamma-receptor gene and susceptibility to mycobacterial infection. New England Journal of Medicine 1996; 335: 1941-1949.
105. Davis EG, Eichenberger MR, Grant BS, Polk HC, Jr. Microsatellite marker of interferon-gamma receptor 1 gene correlates with infection following major trauma. Surgery 2000; 128: 301-305.
106. Beutler B, Poltorak A. The sole gateway to endotoxin response: how LPS was identified as Tlr4, and its role in innate immunity. Drug Metabolism and Disposition 2001; 29: 474-478.
107. Arbour NC, Lorenz E, Schutte BC, et al. TLR4 mutations are associated with endotoxin hyporesponsiveness in humans. Nature Genetics 2000; 25: 187-191.
108. Agnese DM, Calvano JE, Hahm SJ, et al. Human toll-like receptor 4 mutations but not CD14 polymorphisms are associated with an increased risk of gram-negative infections. Journal of Infectious Disease 2002; 186: 1522-1525.
109. Kiechl S, Lorenz E, Reindl M, et al. Toll-like receptor 4 polymorphisms and atherogenesis. New England Journal of Medicine 2002; 347: 185-192.
110. Lorenz E, Mira JP, Frees KL, Schwartz DA. Relevance of mutations in the TLR4 receptor in patients with gram-negative

septic shock. Archives of Internal Medicine 2002; 162: 1028-1032.
111. Child NJ, Yang IA, Pulletz MC, et al. Polymorphisms in Toll-like receptor 4 and the systemic inflammatory response syndrome. Biochemical Society Transactions 2003; 31: 652-653.
112. Tracey KJ, Beutler B, Lowry SF, et al. Shock and tissue injury induced by recombinant human cachectin. Science 1986; 234: 470-474.
113. Stechmiller JK, Treloar D, Allen N. Gut dysfunction in critically ill patients: a review of the literature. American Journal of Critical Care 1997; 6: 204-209.
114. Sutherland AM, Walley KR, Russell JA. Polymorphisms in CD14, mannose-binding lectin, and Toll-like receptor-2 are associated with increased prevalence of infection in critically ill adults. Critical Care Medicine 2005; 33: 638-644.
115. Nakada TA, Hirasawa H, Oda S, et al. Influence of toll-like receptor 4, CD14, tumor necrosis factor, and interleukine-10 gene polymorphisms on clinical outcome in Japanese critically ill patients. Journal of Surgical Research 2005; 129: 322-328.
116. Hubacek JA, Stuber F, Frohlich D, et al. Gene variants of the bactericidal/permeability increasing protein and lipopolysaccharide binding protein in sepsis patients: gender-specific genetic predisposition to sepsis. Critical Care Medicine 2001; 29: 557-561.
117. Barber RC, O'Keefe GE. Characterization of a single nucleotide polymorphism in the lipopolysaccharide binding protein and its association with sepsis. American Journal of Respiratory and Critical Care Medicine 2003; 167: 1316-1320.
118. Garred P, Strom J, Quist L, Taaning E, Madsen HO. Association of mannose-binding lectin polymorphisms with sepsis and fatal outcome, in patients with systemic inflammatory response syndrome. Journal of Infectious Disease 2003; 188: 1394-1403.
119. Schumann RR, Leong SR, Flaggs GW, et al. Structure and function of lipopolysaccharide binding protein. Science 1990; 249: 1429-1431.
120. Weiss J, Muello K, Victor M, Elsbach P. The role of lipopolysaccharides in the action of the bactericidal/permeability-increasing neutrophil protein on the bacterial envelope. Journal of Immunology 1984; 132: 3109-3115.
121. Elsbach P, Weiss J. Role of the bactericidal/permeability-increasing protein in host defence. Current Opinions in Immunology 1998; 10: 45-49.
122. Tobias PS, Soldau K, Iovine NM, Elsbach P, Weiss J. Lipopolysaccharide (LPS)-binding proteins BPI and LBP form

different types of complexes with LPS. Journal of Biological Chemistry 1997; 272: 18682-18685.
123. Ulevitch RJ, Tobias PS. Receptor-dependent mechanisms of cell stimulation by bacterial endotoxin. Annual Review of Immunology 1995; 13: 437-457.
124. Baldini M, Lohman IC, Halonen M, Erickson RP, Holt PG, Martinez FD. A Polymorphism* in the 5' flanking region of the CD14 gene is associated with circulating soluble CD14 levels and with total serum immunoglobulin E. American Journal of Respiratory Cell and Molecular Biology 1999; 20: 976-983.
125. Hubacek JA, Rothe G, Pit'ha J, et al. C(-260)-->T polymorphism in the promoter of the CD14 monocyte receptor gene as a risk factor for myocardial infarction. Circulation 1999; 99: 3218-3220.
126. Unkelbach K, Gardemann A, Kostrzewa M, Philipp M, Tillmanns H, Haberbosch W. A new promoter polymorphism in the gene of lipopolysaccharide receptor CD14 is associated with expired myocardial infarction in patients with low atherosclerotic risk profile. Arteriosclerosis, Thrombosis, and Vascular Biology 1999; 19: 932-938.
127. Ripoll L, Collet JP, Barateau V. A novel CD14 gene polymorphism that determines variable monocyte activation is associated with the risk of myocardial infarction in young adults. Circulation 1999; 18: 1821.
128. Gibot S, Cariou A, Drouet L, Rossignol M, Ripoll L. Association between a genomic polymorphism within the CD14 locus and septic shock susceptibility and mortality rate. Critical Care Medicine 2002; 30: 969-973.
129. Burgmann H, Winkler S, Locker GJ, et al. Increased serum concentration of soluble CD14 is a prognostic marker in gram-positive sepsis. Clinical Immunology and Immunopathology 1996; 80: 307-310.
130. Landmann R, Zimmerli W, Sansano S, et al. Increased circulating soluble CD14 is associated with high mortality in gram-negative septic shock. Journal of Infectious Disease 1995; 171: 639-644.
131. Landmann R, Reber AM, Sansano S, Zimmerli W. Function of soluble CD14 in serum from patients with septic shock. Journal of Infectious Disease 1996; 173: 661-668.
132. Goyert SM, Ferrero E, Rettig WJ, Yenamandra AK, Obata F, Le Beau MM. The CD14 monocyte differentiation antigen maps to a region encoding growth factors and receptors. Science 1988; 239: 497-500.
133. Gong MN, Wei Z, Xu LL, Miller DP, Thompson BT, Christiani DC. Polymorphism in the surfactant protein-B gene, gender, and

the risk of direct pulmonary injury and ARDS. Chest 2004; 125: 203-211.
134. Hermans PW, Hazelzet JA. Plasminogen activator inhibitor type 1 gene polymorphism and sepsis. Clinical Infectious Diseases 2005; 41: S453-S458.
135. Eriksson P, Kallin B, van 't Hooft FM, Bavenholm P, Hamsten A. Allele-specific increase in basal transcription of the plasminogen-activator inhibitor 1 gene is associated with myocardial infarction. Procedings of the National Academy of Science of the USA 1995; 92: 1851-1855.
136. Dawson SJ, Wiman B, Hamsten A, Green F, Humphries S, Henney AM. The two allele sequences of a common polymorphism in the promoter of the plasminogen activator inhibitor-1 (PAI-1) gene respond differently to interleukin-1 in HepG2 cells. Journal of Biological Chemistry 1993; 268: 10739-10745.
137. Menges T, Hermans PW, Little SG, *et al*. Plasminogen-activator-inhibitor-1 4G/5G promoter polymorphism and prognosis of severely injured patients. Lancet 2001; 357: 1096-1097.
138. Biemond BJ, Levi M, Ten Cate H, *et al*. Plasminogen activator and plasminogen activator inhibitor I release during experimental endotoxaemia in chimpanzees: effect of interventions in the cytokine and coagulation cascades. Clinical Science (Lond) 1995; 88: 587-594.
139. Gando S. Disseminated intravascular coagulation in trauma patients. Seminars in Thrombosis and Hemostasis 2001; 27: 585-592.
140. Hazelzet JA, Risseeuw-Appel IM, *et al*. Age-related differences in outcome and severity of DIC in children with septic shock and purpura. Thrombosis and Haemostasis 1996; 76: 932-938.
141. Mesters RM, Florke N, Ostermann H, Kienast J. Increase of plasminogen activator inhibitor levels predicts outcome of leukocytopenic patients with sepsis. Thrombosis and Haemostasis 1996; 75: 902-907.
142. Gando S, Kameue T, Nanzaki S, Nakanishi Y. Disseminated intravascular coagulation is a frequent complication of systemic inflammatory response syndrome. Thrombosis and Haemostasis 1996; 75: 224-228.
143. Nicolaes GA, Dahlback B. Activated protein C resistance (FV(Leiden)) and thrombosis: factor V mutations causing hypercoagulable states. Hematology/Oncology Clinics of North America 2003; 17: 37-61.
144. Kondaveeti S, Hibberd ML, Booy R, Nadel S, Levin M. Effect of the Factor V Leiden mutation on the severity of

meningococcal disease. Pediatric Infectious Disease Journal 1999; 18: 893-896.
145. Kerlin BA, Yan SB, Isermann BH, *et al.* Survival advantage associated with heterozygous factor V Leiden mutation in patients with severe sepsis and in mouse endotoxemia. Blood 2003; 102: 3085-3092.
146. Taylor FB, Jr., Chang A, Hinshaw LB, Esmon CT, Archer LT, Beller BK. A model for thrombin protection against endotoxin. Thrombosis Research 1984; 36: 177-185.
147. Arnaud E, Barbalat V, Nicaud V, *et al.* Polymorphisms in the 5' regulatory region of the tissue factor gene and the risk of myocardial infarction and venous thromboembolism: the ECTIM and PATHROS studies. Etude Cas-Temoins de l'Infarctus du Myocarde. Paris Thrombosis case-control Study. Arteriosclerosis, Thrombosis, and Vascular Biology 2000; 20: 892-898.
148. Weiler H, Lindner V, Kerlin B, *et al.* Characterization of a mouse model for thrombomodulin deficiency. Arteriosclerosis, Thrombosis, and Vascular Biology 2001; 21: 1531-1537.
149. Kottke-Marchant K. Genetic polymorphisms associated with venous and arterial thrombosis: an overview. Archives of Pathology and Laboratory Medicine 2002; 126: 295-304.
150. Medford AR, Keen LJ, Bidwell JL, Millar AB. Vascular endothelial growth factor gene polymorphism and acute respiratory distress syndrome. Thorax 2005; 60: 244-248.
151. Marshall RP, Webb S, Bellingan GJ, *et al.* Angiotensin converting enzyme insertion/deletion polymorphism is associated with susceptibility and outcome in acute respiratory distress syndrome. American Journal of Respiratory and Critical Care Medicine 2002; 166: 646-650.
152. Rigat B, Hubert C, henc-Gelas F, Cambien F, Corvol P, Soubrier F. An insertion/deletion polymorphism in the angiotensin I-converting enzyme gene accounting for half the variance of serum enzyme levels. Journal of Clinical Investigation 1990; 86: 1343-1346.
153. Marshall RP, Webb S, Hill MR, Humphries SE, Laurent GJ. Genetic polymorphisms associated with susceptibility and outcome in ARDS. Chest 2002; 121: 68S-69S.
154. Kiang JG, Tsokos GC. Heat shock protein 70 kDa: molecular biology, biochemistry, and physiology. Pharmacology and Therapeutics 1998; 80: 183-201.
155. Baler R, Zou J, Voellmy R. Evidence for a role of Hsp70 in the regulation of the heat shock response in mammalian cells. Cell Stress & Chaperones 1996; 1: 33-39.

156. Sistonen L, Sarge KD, Morimoto RI. Human heat shock factors 1 and 2 are differentially activated and can synergistically induce hsp70 gene transcription. Molecular and Cellular Biology 1994; 14: 2087-2099.
157. Soncin F, Prevelige R, Calderwood SK. Expression and purification of human heat-shock transcription factor 1. Protein Expression and Purification 1997; 9: 27-32.
158. Asea A, Kraeft SK, Kurt-Jones EA, *et al*. HSP70 stimulates cytokine production through a CD14-dependant pathway, demonstrating its dual role as a chaperone and cytokine. Nature Medicine 2000; 6: 435-442.
159. DeNagel DC, Pierce SK. A case for chaperones in antigen processing. Immunology Today 1992; 13: 86-89.
160. Ribeiro SP, Villar J, Downey GP, Edelson JD, Slutsky AS. Effects of the stress response in septic rats and LPS-stimulated alveolar macrophages: evidence for TNF-alpha posttranslational regulation. American Journal of Respiratory and Critical Care Medicine 1996; 154: 1843-1850.
161. Nishimura H, Emoto M, Kimura K, Yoshikai Y. Hsp70 protects macrophages infected with Salmonella choleraesuis against TNF-alpha-induced cell death. Cell Stress & Chaperones 1997; 2: 50-59.
162. Milner CM, Campbell RD. Structure and expression of the three MHC-linked HSP70 genes. Immunogenetics 1990; 32: 242-251.
163. Hunt C, Morimoto RI. Conserved features of eukaryotic hsp70 genes revealed by comparison with the nucleotide sequence of human hsp70. Procedings of the National Academy of Science of the USA 1985; 82: 6455-6459.
164. Ito Y, Ando A, Ando H, *et al*. Genomic structure of the spermatid-specific hsp70 homolog gene located in the class III region of the major histocompatibility complex of mouse and man. Journal of Biochemistry (Tokyo) 1998; 124: 347-353.
165. Waterer GW, El Bahlawan L, Quasney MW, Zhang Q, Kessler LA, Wunderink RG. Heat shock protein 70-2+1267 AA homozygotes have an increased risk of septic shock in adults with community-acquired pneumonia. Critical Care Medicine 2003; 31: 1367-1372.
166. Favatier F, Bornman L, Hightower LE, Gunther E, Polla BS. Variation in hsp gene expression and Hsp polymorphism: do they contribute to differential disease susceptibility and stress tolerance? Cell Stress & Chaperones 1997; 2: 141-155.
167. Temple SE, Cheong KY, Ardlie KG, Sayer D, Waterer GW. The septic shock associated HSPA1B1267 polymorphism influences production of HSPA1A and HSPA1B. Intensive Care Medicine 2004; 30: 1761-1767.

168. Cohen J. The immunopathogenesis of sepsis. Nature 2002; 420: 885-891.
169. Fraunberger P, Pilz G, Cremer P, Werdan K, Walli AK. Association of serum tumor necrosis factor levels with decrease of cholesterol during septic shock. Shock 1998; 10: 359-363.
170. Gordon BR, Parker TS, Levine DM, *et al.* Relationship of hypolipidemia to cytokine concentrations and outcomes in critically ill surgical patients. Critical Care Medicine 2001; 29: 1563-1568.
171. van Leeuwen HJ, Heezius EC, Dallinga GM, van Strijp JA, Verhoef J, van Kessel KP. Lipoprotein metabolism in patients with severe sepsis. Critical Care Medicine 2003; 31: 1359-1366.
172. Fogelman AM. When good cholesterol goes bad. Nature Medicine 2004; 10: 902-903.
173. Chenaud C, Merlani PG, Roux-Lombard P, *et al.* Low apolipoprotein A-I level at intensive care unit admission and systemic inflammatory response syndrome exacerbation. Critical Care Medicine 2004; 32: 632-637.
174. Levels JH, Lemaire LC, van den Ende AE, van Deventer SJ, van Lanschot JJ. Lipid composition and lipopolysaccharide binding capacity of lipoproteins in plasma and lymph of patients with systemic inflammatory response syndrome and multiple organ failure. Critical Care Medicine 2003; 31: 1647-1653.
175. de BN, Netea MG, Demacker PN, Verschueren I, *et al.* Apolipoprotein E knock-out mice are highly susceptible to endotoxemia and Klebsiella pneumoniae infection. Journal of Lipid Research 1999; 40: 680-685.
176. Roselaar SE, Daugherty A. Apolipoprotein E-deficient mice have impaired innate immune responses to Listeria monocytogenes in vivo. Journal of Lipid Research 1998; 39: 1740-1743.
177. Vonk AG, de BN, Netea MG, *et al.* Apolipoprotein-E-deficient mice exhibit an increased susceptibility to disseminated candidiasis. Medical Mycology 2004; 42: 341-348.
178. Lynch JR, Morgan D, Mance J, Matthew WD, Laskowitz DT. Apolipoprotein E modulates glial activation and the endogenous central nervous system inflammatory response. Journal of Neuroimmunology 2001; 114: 107-113.
179. Van Oosten M, Rensen PC, Van Amersfoort ES, *et al.* Apolipoprotein E protects against bacterial lipopolysaccharide-induced lethality. A new therapeutic approach to treat gram-negative sepsis. Journal of Biological Chemistry 2001; 276: 8820-8824.

180. Guo L, LaDu MJ, Van Eldik LJ. A dual role for apolipoprotein e in neuroinflammation: anti- and pro-inflammatory activity. Journal of Molecular Neuroscience 2004; 23: 205-212.
181. Mahley RW, Rall SC, Jr. Apolipoprotein E: far more than a lipid transport protein. Annual Review of Genomics and Human Genetics 2000; 1: 507-537.
182. Bohnet K, Pillot T, Visvikis S, Sabolovic N, Siest G. Apolipoprotein (apo) E genotype and apoE concentration determine binding of normal very low density lipoproteins to HepG2 cell surface receptors. Journal of Lipid Research 1996; 37: 1316-1324.
183. Mamotte CD, Sturm M, Foo JI, van Bockxmeer FM, Taylor RR. Comparison of the LDL-receptor binding of VLDL and LDL from apoE4 and apoE3 homozygotes. American Journal of Physiology 1999; 276: E553-E557.
184. Moretti EW, Morris RW, Podgoreanu M, *et al*. APOE polymorphism is associated with risk of severe sepsis in surgical patients. Critical Care Medicine 2005; 33: 2521-2526.
185. Baugh JA, Bucala R. Macrophage migration inhibitory factor. Critical Care Medicine 2002; 30: S27-S35.
186. Calandra T, Bernhagen J, Metz CN, *et al*. MIF as a glucocorticoid-induced modulator of cytokine production. Nature 1995; 377: 68-71.
187. Lue H, Kleemann R, Calandra T, Roger T, Bernhagen J. Macrophage migration inhibitory factor (MIF): mechanisms of action and role in disease. Microbes and Infection 2002; 4: 449-460.
188. Bernhagen J, Calandra T, Mitchell RA, *et al*. MIF is a pituitary-derived cytokine that potentiates lethal endotoxaemia. Nature 1993; 365: 756-759.
189. Calandra T, Spiegel LA, Metz CN, Bucala R. Macrophage migration inhibitory factor is a critical mediator of the activation of immune cells by exotoxins of Gram-positive bacteria. Procedings of the National Academy of Science of the USA 1998; 95: 11383-11388.
190. Beishuizen A, Thijs LG, Haanen C, Vermes I. Macrophage migration inhibitory factor and hypothalamo-pituitary-adrenal function during critical illness. Journal of Clinical Endocrinology and Metabolism 2001; 86: 2811-2816.
191. Bozza FA, Gomes RN, Japiassu AM, *et al*. Macrophage migration inhibitory factor levels correlate with fatal outcome in sepsis. Shock 2004; 22: 309-313.
192. Gando S, Nishihira J, Kobayashi S, Morimoto Y, Nanzaki S, Kemmotsu O. Macrophage migration inhibitory factor is a

critical mediator of systemic inflammatory response syndrome. Intensive Care Medicine 2001; 27: 1187-1193.
193. De Benedetti F, Meazza C, Vivarelli M, et al. Functional and prognostic relevance of the -173 polymorphism of the macrophage migration inhibitory factor gene in systemic-onset juvenile idiopathic arthritis. Arthritis and Rheumatism 2003; 48: 1398-1407.
194. Donn R, Alourfi Z, De BF, et al. Mutation screening of the macrophage migration inhibitory factor gene: positive association of a functional polymorphism of macrophage migration inhibitory factor with juvenile idiopathic arthritis. Arthritis and Rheumatism 2002; 46: 2402-2409.
195. Donn RP, Shelley E, Ollier WE, Thomson W. A novel 5'-flanking region polymorphism of macrophage migration inhibitory factor is associated with systemic-onset juvenile idiopathic arthritis. Arthritis and Rheumatism 2001; 44: 1782-1785.
196. Wang JE. Can single nucleotide polymorphisms in innate immune receptors predict development of septic complications in intensive care unit patients? Critical Care Medicine 2005; 33: 695-696.
197. Bernard GR, Vincent JL, Laterre PF, et al. Efficacy and safety of recombinant human activated protein C for severe sepsis. New England Journal of Medicine 2001; 344: 699-709.
198. Rivers E, Nguyen B, Havstad S, et al. Early goal-directed therapy in the treatment of severe sepsis and septic shock. New England Journal of Medicine 2001; 345: 1368-1377.
199. Rivers EP, Nguyen HB, Huang DT, Donnino M. Early goal-directed therapy. Critical Care Medicine 2004; 32: 314-315.
200. Rivers EP. Early goal-directed therapy in severe sepsis and septic shock: converting science to reality. Chest 2006; 129: 217-218.
201. Vincent JL, Sun Q, Dubois MJ. Clinical trials of immunomodulatory therapies in severe sepsis and septic shock. Clinical Infectious Diseases 2002; 34: 1084-1093.
202. Dahabreh Z, Dimitriou R, Chalidis B, Giannoudis PV. Coagulopathy and the role of recombinant human activated protein C in sepsis and following polytrauma. Expert Opinion on Drug Safety 2006; 5: 67-82.
203. Harding D, Baines PB, Brull D, et al. Severity of meningococcal disease in children and the angiotensin-converting enzyme insertion/deletion polymorphism. American Journal of Respiratory and Critical Care Medicine 2002; 165: 1103-1106.
204. Hubacek JA, Stuber F, Frohlich D, et al. The common functional C(-159)T polymorphism within the promoter region

of the lipopolysaccharide receptor CD14 is not associated with sepsis development or mortality. Genes and Immunity 2000; 1: 405-407.
205. Schroeder S, Reck M, Hoeft A, Stuber F. Analysis of two human leukocyte antigen-linked polymorphic heat shock protein 70 genes in patients with severe sepsis. Critical Care Medicine 1999; 27: 1265-1270.
206. Schroder O, Schulte KM, Ostermann P, Roher HD, Ekkernkamp A, Laun RA. Heat shock protein 70 genotypes HSPA1B and HSPA1L influence cytokine concentrations and interfere with outcome after major injury. Critical Care Medicine 2003; 31: 73-79.
207. Madsen HO, Garred P, Thiel S, *et al*. Interplay between promoter and structural gene variants control basal serum level of mannan-binding protein. Journal of Immunology 1995; 155: 3013-3020.
208. Sumiya M, Super M, Tabona P, *et al*. Molecular basis of opsonic defect in immunodeficient children. Lancet 1991; 337: 1569-1570.
209. Super M, Thiel S, Lu J, Levinsky RJ, Turner MW. Association of low levels of mannan-binding protein with a common defect of opsonisation. Lancet 1989; 2: 1236-1239.
210. Westendorp RG, Hottenga JJ, Slagboom PE. Variation in plasminogen-activator-inhibitor-1 gene and risk of meningococcal septic shock. Lancet 1999; 354: 561-563.
211. Geishofer G, Binder A, Muller M, *et al*. 4G/5G promoter polymorphism in the plasminogen-activator-inhibitor-1 gene in children with systemic meningococcaemia. European Journal of Pediatrics 2005; 164: 486-490.
212. Hermans PW, Hibberd ML, Booy R, *et al*. 4G/5G promoter polymorphism in the plasminogen-activator-inhibitor-1 gene and outcome of meningococcal disease. Meningococcal Research Group. Lancet 1999; 354: 556-560.
213. Ogus AC, Yoldas B, Ozdemir T, *et al*. The Arg753GLn polymorphism of the human toll-like receptor 2 gene in tuberculosis disease. European Respiratory Journal 2004; 23: 219-223.
214. Lorenz E, Mira JP, Cornish KL, Arbour NC, Schwartz DA. A novel polymorphism in the toll-like receptor 2 gene and its potential association with staphylococcal infection. Infection and Immunity 2000; 68: 6398-6401.
215. Feterowski C, Emmanuilidis K, Miethke T, *et al*. Effects of functional Toll-like receptor-4 mutations on the immune response to human and experimental sepsis. Immunology 2003; 109: 426-431.

216. Nadel S, Newport MJ, Booy R, Levin M. Variation in the tumor necrosis factor-alpha gene promoter region may be associated with death from meningococcal disease. Journal of Infectious Disease 1996; 174: 878-880.
217. Waterer GW, Quasney MW, Cantor RM, Wunderink RG. Septic shock and respiratory failure in community-acquired pneumonia have different TNF polymorphism associations. American Journal of Respiratory and Critical Care Medicine 2001; 163: 1599-1604.

12: Low Volume versus High Volume Resuscitation in Trauma

PROF MONTY MYTHEN

Introduction
Traumatic injury is one of the commonest causes of death in the world irrespective of national wealth or health. According to a World Health Organisation report published in 2002, there are an estimated 5 million deaths from trauma per annum (equating to 8.3/100,000 population) representing 9% of worldwide deaths and 12% of the overall disease burden [1]. Road traffic injury contributed to 1.2 million deaths per annum (ranked 11th commonest cause of death) and somewhere between 20 and 50 million injuries. The mechanisms of injury leading to death are quite variable but central nervous system injury (especially head injury) is the leading overall cause of death (40-50% of trauma associated deaths) followed by traumatic haemorrhage (30-40%) [2].

Resuscitation
Successful resuscitation from traumatic haemorrhage requires early restoration of the heart-lung-brain circulation to avoid immediate death; however, complete restoration of the circulation must follow to allow long term survival. As little as 50% replacement of blood volume is all that may be required to restore a viable heart-lung-brain circulation in non-anaesthetised, non-sedated humans but at least 100% of blood volume will need to be restored to re-perfuse all organs, especially the splanchnic bed [2,3].

Trauma resuscitation can be divided into four phases: early pre-hospital (the field), resuscitative (the emergency room), operative (the operating theatre) and critical care. Traumatic haemorrhage may be further classified as surgical (i.e. can be stopped by pressing, clamping or suturing) or non-surgical [2].

Early pre-hospital resuscitation of traumatic haemorrhage presents a dilemma. Definitive control of bleeding is often not possible. Inadequate resuscitation will contribute to mortality but restoration of the circulation prior to haemostasis may result in further haemorrhage and death. Broadly, there are two schools of field resuscitation "scoop and run" or "stay and play". The "scoop and run" school favours minimal resuscitation (i.e. aims to restore a palpable pulse) followed by immediate transfer to a medical facility. Proponents of "stay and play" maintain that full resuscitation of the circulation should be a primary goal in the field and that this may necessitate immediate control of surgical bleeding (e.g. thoracotomy or laparotomy). Clearly such control requires a high level of field surgical skill.

Resuscitation fluid
However for both schools of thought, there is the choice of resuscitation fluid: colloid versus crystalloid, iso-osmolar/ -oncotic versus hyper-osmolar/ -oncotic, saline versus Lactated Ringer's [3-8]. Current opinion, based on animal and limited human studies, supports a strategy of 'hypotensive resuscitation' in the pre-hospital phase with an isotonic crystalloid (e.g. Lactated Ringer's or Hartmann's solutions). In the UK, the consensus view of experienced trauma personnel on pre-hospital fluid resuscitation in traumatic haemorrhage was published in the Emergency Medicine Journal in 2002 [9]. They concluded that:

> "Fluids should not be administered to trauma victims before haemorrhage control if a radial pulse can be felt. Judicious aliquots of 250 ml [of isotonic crystalloid] should be titrated for other patients. If the radial pulse returns, fluid resuscitation can be suspended for the present and the situation monitored. In penetrating torso trauma, the presence of a central pulse should be considered adequate. In children less than 1 year old, the use of a brachial pulse is more practical as it is easier to feel."

The evidence base for the statement is animal studies, expert opinion and a single centre randomised control trial. This trial was originally published in the New England Journal of Medicine in 1994 by Bickell *et al.* [10]. A recent review of progress in intensive care medicine in the past 25 years highlighted this study as the only adequate trial in multiple trauma victims [11].

Bickell and others at the Ben Taub General Hospital in Houston, USA conducted a prospective trial comparing immediate and delayed fluid resuscitation in 598 adults with penetrating torso injuries who presented with a pre-hospital systolic blood pressure of ≤ 90 mmHg [10]. Patients eligible for the study were adults or adolescents (>16 years) with stab or gunshot wounds to the torso. Following initial on-scene assessment and treatment by paramedics from The City of Houston Medical Services all patients were ground transferred to the city's only trauma hospital. A policy of waived consent, adhering to the principle of implied consent was used. In all patients surgery was only performed in hospital. Patients were assigned to either receive immediate-resuscitation in which fluid was given before surgery, or delayed-resuscitation where no fluid was given until the time of surgery. Surgery included thoracotomy, laparotomy, neck and groin exploration.

Patients randomised to the immediate-resuscitation group had two or more 14 gauge intravenous cannulae placed in their upper extremities and were infused with isotonic Ringer's acetate *en-route* to hospital. Patients with a systolic arterial pressure of less than 100 mmHg on arrival at the trauma centre received a continuous infusion of Ringer's acetate. Blood and blood products were transfused according to national guidelines. Patients randomised to the delayed group received identical treatment but following the insertion of the cannulae they were capped and flushed. The main outcome variable was survival to hospital discharge. The study was powered to detect a 10-15% difference in mortality assuming a mortality rate in the immediate resuscitation group of 35%.

Table 1. Difference in fluid requirements (means ± standard deviations) between patients with immediate and delayed resuscitation (*: $p < 0.05$).

VARIABLE	IMMEDIATE RESUSCITATION (N = 309)	DELAYED RESUSCITATION (N = 289)
Before arrival at the hospital		
Ringer's acetate; ml	870±667	92±309*
Trauma centre		
Ringer's acetate; ml	1608±1201	283±722*
Packed red cells; ml	133 ±393	11 ±88*
Operating room		
Ringer's acetate; ml	6772±4688	6529±4863
Packed red cells; ml	1942±2322	1713±2313
Fresh-frozen plasma or platelet packs; ml	357±1002	307±704
Autologous-transfusion volume; ml	95±486	111 ±690
Hetastarch; ml	499±717	542±696
Rate of intra-operative fluid administration; ml/min	117±126	91±88*

CRITICAL CARE FOCUS 14: UPDATES

The immediate resuscitation group received an average 2,103 ml extra of Ringer's acetate compared to the delayed resuscitation group (2,478 versus 375 ml) prior to surgery (Table 1). On arrival at the trauma centre the delayed resuscitation group had slightly lower average systolic blood pressure (72 versus 79 mmHg), higher haemoglobin and platelet counts and more normal coagulation parameters (Table 2). At study completion the mortality rate prior to hospital discharge was higher in the immediate-resuscitation group (38% versus 30%, p = 0.04).

Table 2. Difference in cardiovascular, coagulation and metabolic parameters (means ± standard deviations) between patients with immediate and delayed resuscitation (*: $p < 0.05$).

VARIABLE	IMMEDIATE RESUSCITATION (N = 309)	DELAYED RESUSCITATION (N = 289)
Systolic blood pressure; mmHg	76±46	72±43*
Haemoglobin; g/dl	11.2±2.6	12.9±2.2*
Platelet count; $x10^3/mm^3$	274±84	297±88*
Prothrombin time; sec	14.1 ±1.6	11.4±1.8*
Partial-thromboplastin time; sec	31.8±19.3	27.5±12.0
Systemic arterial pH	7.29±0.17	7.28±0.15
Serum bicarbonate; mmol/l	20±10	20±11

When using this study to guide current UK practice, it is important to note the following. This was a single centre study conducted between 1989 and 1992 by paramedics delivering patients to a dedicated trauma centre in the USA. More than 85% of the study subjects were young males with a mean age of 30 yrs. Approximately 70% had been shot and 30% stabbed in the torso. Patients with significant head injury were excluded. Total times from call to arrival in the trauma centre were on average < 30 mins including response, initial treatment at scene and transfer. The subjects were treated with Ringer's acetate (not Ringer's lactate or normal saline). Although it is unlikely that the use of an acetate buffered isotonic crystalloid solution rather than the more commonly available lactate buffered solutions (Ringer's lactate or Hartmann's solution) or isotonic 0.9% sodium chloride solution would have materially altered the main outcomes this point is worthy of note. In the UK, most trauma is blunt and there is little evidence from human studies of the differences one might expect with blunt rather than penetrating trauma. Blunt trauma commonly involves more contusion of internal organs including the brain and risk of swelling in confined spaces whereas penetrating trauma is more commonly associated with brisk haemorrhage from cut vessels. Dutton *et al.* [4] randomised 110 patients who had suffered penetrating and / or blunt trauma to standard resuscitation or treatment by according to an algorithm where fluid was titrated to achieve a systolic blood pressure of 70-80 mmHg. In this small study, there was no difference in mortality between the two groups but the overall mortality was only 7% so the study was grossly underpowered.

Hospital phase (emergency room, operating theatre and critical care)
The emergency room phase is a continuum from the field but with an increase in availability of expertise and equipment. Accepting the fact that if low volume or minimal resuscitation is beneficial, it can only be tolerated for a short duration and must be followed by prompt attention to haemorrhage control and full resuscitation with colloids, blood and blood products. The key is the time to control of surgical haemorrhage. This is achieved very rapidly in countries with effective retrieval services, para-medic or doctor led field resuscitation teams and dedicated trauma centres [6, 7]. If trauma patients are received by non-specialist centres, then the small amount of evidence from human studies is even harder to interpret and apply but once surgical bleeding is controlled then the best available evidence based approach to further resuscitation is the same as any other critically ill patient. The aim is to restore a full circulation and optimal perfusion of all tissues guided by appropriate monitoring. Early goal directed therapy aiming to restore routinely measured haemodynamic variables and surrogates of tissue oxygenation (e.g. central venous saturation, base deficit and lactate) is generally thought to produce long term benefits but there is limited data from trauma studies to support this [12]. In choosing the type of fluid all commonly available choices have putative benefits and risks. Colloids are more efficient at restoring the intravascular volume and should cause less oedema but they are more expensive than crystalloids (although in reality very cheap); however they may exacerbate coagulopathy. Crystalloids are considerably less expensive per unit volume but are also less efficient at restoring the intravascular space and can cause clinically significant oedema (e.g. abdominal compartment syndrome). Normal (0.9%) saline causes hyperchloraemia and acidosis which may result in renal dysfunction, reduced gastro-intestinal tract perfusion. Lactated Ringer's contains calcium which may prevent its co-administration with citrated blood and lactate which will elevate serum lactate levels (but not cause an

acidosis) so causing diagnostic confusion. Furthermore, lactated Ringer's is relatively hypotonic which may exacerbate cerebral oedema following traumatic brain injury. Blood and blood products are very expensive and not always immediately available but are a key early component of restoring an adequate oxygen delivery and correcting coagulopathy [12,13]. It is generally accepted that a higher transfusion trigger (e.g. 10 g/dl) is a reasonable one for resuscitation rather than the 7 g/dl more commonly used for the longer term ICU patient. This will need to be adjusted according to degree of ongoing haemorrhage and success in achieving resuscitation goals. Once again there is little evidence from adequately powered well designed clinical trials to allow evidence based recommendations.

The SAFE study of nearly 7,000 critically ill patients randomised patients admitted to intensive care to either albumin or normal saline for volume resuscitation and included a sub-set of 1,186 trauma patients [14,17]. Patients randomised to receive albumin experienced significantly greater mortality associated with a higher incidence of intra-cerebral bleeding. Although the study was not designed to address this specific question, these findings have reinforced the existing recommendation that isotonic crystalloid should be the resuscitation fluid of choice both in the field and early in hospital care until a significant head injury has been ruled out [9]. It is hard to see any role for albumin but the combination commonly used in the UK of lactated Ringer's for hydration and a synthetic colloid (e.g. a 130/0.4 starch) for volume resuscitation remains a logical choice in non-head injured patients. There is certainly no evidence to support a change from this practice.

Hypertonic and hyperoncotic solutions have theoretical advantages supported by animal data in early trauma resuscitation, particularly when there is closed head injury [2,15]. However, no human study has demonstrated a clear positive effect on outcome. Even so many trauma centres now use small volumes of hypertonic and hyperoncotic solutions for early resuscitation particularly if there is a head injury. Perflurocarbons and stroma-free haemoglobin solutions remain experimental products. A European multi-centre trial of a stroma free haemoglobin solution, Diasprin Cross-Linked Haemoglobin (DCLHb) was stopped following recruitment of 112 patients due to excess mortality in the patients who received DCLHb (46% versus 17% respectively, p= 0.003).

Conclusion
Accepting that there is very little evidence from adequately designed human trials, best available evidence supports the following approach

to trauma resuscitation. In the field, the aim is to restore a pulse with boluses of isotonic crystalloid and transfer to hospital should not be delayed. Once surgical haemorrhage is controlled and a significant head injury has been excluded then lactated Ringer's can be used for hydration and a synthetic colloid used to restore intravascular volume as guided by appropriate monitoring. Blood and blood products will be needed and should be given early. In patients with traumatic brain injury, normal saline remains the fluid of choice for early resuscitation.

References

1. Peden M, McGee K, Sharma G. The Injury Chart Book: a Graphical Overview of the Global Burden of Injuries. Geneva: World Health Organization, 2002.
2. Kauvar DS, Wade CE. The epidemiology and modern management of traumatic hemorrhage: US and international perspectives. Critical Care 2005; 9: S1-S9.
3. Blow O, Magliore L, Claridge JA, Butler K, Young JS. The golden hour and the silver day: detection and correction of occult hypoperfusion within 24 hours improves outcome from major trauma. Journal of Trauma 1999; 4: 964-969.
4. Dutton RP, Mackenzie CF, Scalea TM. Hypotensive resuscitation during active hemorrhage: impact on in-hospital mortality. Journal of Trauma 2002; 52: 1141-1146.
5. Wears RL, Winton CN. Load and go versus stay and play: analysis of prehospital i.v. fluid therapy by computer simulation. Annals of Emergency Medicine 1990; 19: 163-168.
6. Demetriades D, Chan L, Cornwell E, *et al*. Paramedic vs private transportation of trauma patients. Effect on outcome. Archives of Surgery 1996; 131: 133-138.
7. Veech RL. Immediate versus delayed fluid resuscitation in patients with trauma. New England Journal of Medicine 1995; 332: 681-682.
8. Chudnofsky CR, Dronen SC, Syverud SA, Hedges JR, Zink BJ. Early versus late fluid resuscitation: lack of effect in porcine hemorrhagic shock. Annals of Emergency Medicine 1989; 18: 122-126.
9. Revell M, Porter K, Greaves I. Fluid resuscitation in prehospital trauma care: a consensus view. Emergency Medicine Journal 2002; 19: 494-498.
10. Bickell WH, Wall MJ, Jr., Pepe PE, *et al*. Immediate versus delayed fluid resuscitation for hypotensive patients with penetrating torso injuries. New England Journal of Medicine 1994; 331: 1105-1109.

11. Vincent JL, Fink MP, Marini JJ, *et al*. Intensive care and emergency medicine: progress over the past 25 years. Chest 2006; 129: 1061-1067.
12. Vercueil A, Grocott MP, Mythen MG. Physiology, pharmacology, and rationale for colloid administration for the maintenance of effective hemodynamic stability in critically ill patients. Transfusion Medicine Reviews 2005; 19: 93-109.
13. Choi PT, Yip G, Quinonez LG, Cook DJ. Crystalloids vs. colloids in fluid resuscitation: a systematic review. Critical Care Medicine 1999; 27: 200-210.
14. Finfer S, Bellomo R, Boyce N, French J, Myburgh J, Norton R. A comparison of albumin and saline for fluid resuscitation in the intensive care unit. New England Journal of Medicine 2004; 350: 2247-2256.
15. Wade CE, Grady JJ, Kramer GC, Younes RN, Gehlsen K, Holcroft JW. Individual patient cohort analysis of the efficacy of hypertonic saline/dextran in patients with traumatic brain injury and hypotension. Journal of Trauma 1997; 42: S61-S65.
16. Sloan EP, Koenigsberg M, Gens D, *et al*. Diaspirin cross-linked hemoglobin (DCLHb) in the treatment of severe traumatic hemorrhagic shock: a randomized controlled efficacy trial. Journal of the American Medical Association 1999; 282: 1857-1864.
17. SAFE Study Investigators; Australian and New Zealand Intensive Care Society Clinical Trials Group; Australian Red Cross Blood Service; George Institute for International Health, Myburgh J, Cooper J, Finfer S, Bellomo R, Norton R, Bishop N, Kai Lo S, Vallance S. Saline or albumin for fluid resuscitation in patients with traumatic brain injury. New England Journal of Medicine 2007; 357: 874-884.